OSCE Questions for the Prin

OSCE Questions for the Primary FRCA

Edited by

Chris Whiten
Consultant Anaesthetist, Imperial College NHS Trust, London, UK

Lara Coppel
ST7 Anaesthetic Registrar, Imperial School of Anaesthesia, London, UK

Abigail Richardson
ST7 Anaesthetic Registrar, Imperial School of Anaesthesia, London, UK

Harriet Kemp
Clinical Research Fellow, Pain Research Group, Imperial College, London, UK

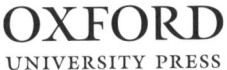

OXFORD
UNIVERSITY PRESS

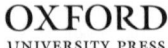
OXFORD
UNIVERSITY PRESS

Great Clarendon Street, Oxford, OX2 6DP,
United Kingdom

Oxford University Press is a department of the University of Oxford.
It furthers the University's objective of excellence in research, scholarship,
and education by publishing worldwide. Oxford is a registered trade mark of
Oxford University Press in the UK and in certain other countries

© Oxford University Press 2016

The moral rights of the authors have been asserted

Impression: 1

Published in the United States of America by Oxford University Press
198 Madison Avenue, New York, NY 10016, United States of America

British Library Cataloguing in Publication Data

Data available

ISBN 978–0–19–875306–3

Printed and bound by CPI Group (UK) Ltd, Croydon, CR0 4YY

Foreword

The Primary FRCA is one of the toughest professional medical examinations in existence. The successful candidate needs to amass a huge amount of knowledge, with a strong emphasis on basic sciences, as well as facing the examiners in person during the OSCE and viva sections of the exam.

When I sat the Primary, more than twelve years ago, I underestimated the OSCE and this is not uncommon as many candidates see it as the easiest part of the exam. This could not be further from the truth! The physical pressures of having to move from station to station, coupled with the need to mentally jump from topic to topic can be incredibly taxing and make it difficult to perform to the best of one's abilities. Preparation is everything, and this can be almost as difficult as the OSCE itself. The idea for this book arose from the experiences of three anaesthetists all of whom had had similar experiences of the OSCE part of the Primary FRCA, and felt that a comprehensive book would be a useful tool to aid preparation for the exam.

Abi, Harriet and Lara devised the concept for this book and set about writing it with the memory of the Primary still fresh in their minds. They have used their collective experiences and knowledge to shape the content of this book, including offering useful tips and advice to prospective Primary candidates. The questions and stations encountered in the book are all typical of those that make up the actual OSCE and they not only offer the chance to practise technique, but also to revise commonly tested knowledge. This book will be invaluable to all doctors attempting the Primary FRCA and also to those more senior anaesthetists involved in helping others to prepare.

Christopher Whiten
October 2015

Contents

Abbreviations

ABC	airway, breathing, circulation
A&E	accident and emergency
AAGBI	The Association of Anaesthatists in Great Britain and Ireland
AS	aortic stenosis
AAS	antlanto-axial subluxation
AF	atrial fibrillation
ALS	amyotrophic lateral sclerosis
AP	anterior-posterior
APL	adjustable pressure limiting
ARDS	acute respiratory distress syndrome
ATLS	advanced trauma life support
AV node	atrioventricular node
BMI	body mass index
BP	blood pressure
bpm	beats per minute
CK	creatine kinase
CSF	cerebrospinal fluid
CMV	cytomegalovirus
CN Va	frontal, lacrimal and nasociliary branches
CN VIII	vestibulocochlear nerve (auditory vestibular nerve), known as the eighth cranial nerve
CN	cranial nerve
COPD	chronic obstructive pulmonary disease
COSHH	control of substances hazardous to health
CPAP	continuous positive airway pressure
CPR	cardiopulmonary resuscitation
CSF	cerebrospinal fluid
CT	computerised axial tomography scan (CAT scan)
CXR	chest X-ray
DC	direct current
DHS	demographic health survey
DMARDS	disease-modifying anti-rheumatic drugs
DOH	Department of Health
ECHO	extended care health option
ECG	electrocardiogram
EEG	electroencephalogram
EMG	electromyogram
EMLA cream	eutetic mixture of local anaesthetics
ENT	ear, nose and throat
FESS	fiberoptic endoscopic sinus surgery
ETA	estimated time of arrival
ETT	exercise tolerance testing
FEV1	forced expiratory volume in 1 second
FRCA	Fellowship of the Royal College of Anaesthetists
FVC	forced vital capacity
GCS	Glasgow coma scale
GFR	glomerular filtration rate

GP	general practitioner
HbA1c l	glycated haemoglobin
HDU	high dependency unit
HELLP	Haemolysis, Elevated Liver enzymes, Low Platelets
Hep B	hepatitis B
Hep C	hepatitis C
HIV	human immunodeficiency virus
HR	heart rate
ICD	implantable cardioverter-defibrillator
ICP	Intracranial pressure
ID	internal diameter of endotracheal tube
IV	intravenous
IgE	immunoglobulin E
IM	intramuscular injection
INR	international normalized ratio
IO	intraosseous
ITU	intensive therapy unit
IUGR	intra-uterine growth retardation
IV	intravenous
JVP	jugular venous pressure
LASER	light amplification by stimulated emission of radiation
LMA	laryngeal mask airway
LMWH	low-molecular-weight heparin
MAP	mean arterial pressure
MI	myocardial infarction
MRI	magnetic resonance imaging
NICE	National Institute for Health and Clinical Excellence
NIBP	noninvasive blood pressure
NIV	non-invasive ventilation
NSAID	nonsteroidal anti-inflammatory drugs
OPSI	overwhelming post-splenectomy infection
OSA	obstructive sleep apnoea
OSCE	objective structured clinical examination
P	systolic Blood Pressure
PA	posterior-anterior
PCA	principal component analysis
PDPH	post-dural-puncture headache
PONV	postoperative nausea and vomiting
PRST	Evans score, simple score used to measure depth of anaesthesia
QRS	combination of three of the graphical deflections seen on a typical electrocardiogram
QRS	quick release system
R	heart Rate
RAE	Ring, Adair, Elwyn
S	Sweating
SI	International System of Units
SOE	Structured Oral Examination
'STOP BANG'	The acronym stands for: S - snoring, T - tiredness during the day, O - observed cessation of breathing, P - high blood Pressure, B - BMI >35, A - Age >50 years old, N - neck circumference >40cm, G - gender (male).
SVC	superior vena cava

Abbreviations

T	Tears
TDS	three times daily
TENS	transcutaneous electrical nerve stimulation
THR	total hip replacement
TIA	transient ischaemic attack
TIVA	total intravenous anaesthesia
TNFα	tumour necrosis factor alpha
TURP	transurethral resection of prostate
VVI	ventricle paced and sensed inhibited

Contributors

James H Briggs,
Consultant Radiologist, Royal Berkshire Hospital, Reading, UK

Alison Carter,
ST7 Anaesthetic Registrar, Imperial School of Anaesthesia, London, UK

Olivia Clancy,
ST5 Anaesthetic Registrar, Imperial School of Anaesthesia, London, UK

Lara Coppel,
ST7 Anaesthetic Registrar, Imperial School of Anaesthesia, London, UK

Betsy Dwyer,
Consultant Anaesthetist, Wexham Park Hospital, Slough, UK

Harriet Kemp,
Clinical Research Fellow, Pain Research Group, Imperial College, London, UK

Abigail Richardson,
ST7 Anaesthetic Registrar, Imperial School of Anaesthesia, London, UK

Chris Whiten,
Consultant Anaesthetist, Imperial College NHS Trust, London,

Introduction

Eighteen stations in one hour and 48 minutes - that is a lot of examination in a relatively short time! The Objective Structured Clinical Examination, or OSCE, has become a common method for assessing undergraduates in medicine and its use in professional examinations was pioneered by the Royal College of Anaesthetists. As its name suggests this section of the Primary FRCA examination is intended to be both objective and structured; meaning that all candidates (on a particular day) are assessed using exactly the same stations, the same marking scheme, and face a range of structured stations that aim to test a large part of the examination curriculum in a fair manner.

To be eligible for entry to the OSCE/ Structured Oral Examination (SOE) part of the Primary FRCA one must have a valid pass in the Primary MCQ and hold an Initial Assessment of Competency Certificate in Anaesthesia. Both the OSCE and SOE must be passed to complete the Primary FRCA. A pass in one or other section, however, is valid for three years and a maximum of six attempts is allowed at this part of the examination.

The range of stations that makes up the Primary FRCA OSCE is predictable and is taken from the basic level curriculum. Sixteen of the eighteen stations count towards the result of the OSCE, with two 'test' stations being included on the day; the 'test' stations are included to trial new questions and both examiners and candidates will NOT know which stations these are. The stations of the OSCE aim to assess candidates on resuscitation (based on 2010 ALS guidelines), technical skills, anatomy (general procedure), history taking, physical examination, communication skills, anaesthetic hazards, and X-ray interpretation. Simulation (medium-fidelity) may be utilised during the OSCE. ALL of the stations must be attempted in order to pass the OSCE.

Each OSCE station lasts for five minutes and starts after a one minute period at an 'information point' prior to entering the station itself. Timings are signaled using a bell, with a double bell used to signal the end of the whole OSCE. It will be evident that this can be incredibly stressful! Candidates have to 'jump' mentally from station to station, and it can be difficult to put a bad experience out of one's mind before starting another station.

Obviously success in the OSCE comes down to achieving sufficient marks to pass! Marking is based on the Angoff method, where the examiners decide the pass mark for each station and each station is marked out of 20. The pass mark for each of the sixteen examination stations is summed to create the overall pass mark for the OSCE, and candidates have to achieve a TOTAL mark that is sufficient to pass. This means it is vital for candidates to treat each station as a fresh part of the exam and not to give up hope if they have had a bad experience; it is possible to pass the OSCE overall even after performing badly in some of the stations. (I can personally vouch for this fact!)

The OSCE requires a different approach and technique to any other form of clinical examination, and focused preparation is invaluable. It can be frustrating and time-consuming to study for the Primary OSCE due to the huge amount of knowledge required and the lack of available resources aimed at this part of the exam. Valuable time may be spent trying to gather all of the information needed to revise effectively, or large sums of money spent on attending OSCE revision courses. This was the reason for the development of this book; it is intended to give the reader a single resource containing commonly occurring types of question along with answers and tips from the authors, aimed at maximising chances of success.

This book is aimed at those candidates looking to familiarise themselves with both the format of the questions/stations they will encounter and the way in which the stations are marked, but also as a way of revising some common topics that often appear in this section of the Primary FRCA examination. It is best used as a 'workbook' with the reader attempting each 'station' before comparing their answers with those given in the book. It is also worth keeping to the time limit that will be imposed for each question in the real exam, as this will help to simulate the stresses faced on the day.

There is a vast amount of knowledge that is needed to pass the Primary FRCA, but candidates often underestimate the OSCE, which can lead to disaster. This book aims to provide a novel and useful way to prepare oneself for the OSCE, both in terms of the format of the questions, common topics encountered and also by covering much of the syllabus of the Primary FRCA. I only wish it had existed back in 2003!

Best of luck!

Christopher Whiten
October 2015

Chapter 1 **Anatomy**

Introduction

There are two anatomy stations in the OSCE. These stations aim to test candidates' knowledge of any anatomical areas associated with common anaesthetic procedures, such as intubation, central and peripheral venous access and nerve blockade. In addition, anatomical knowledge of the cardiovascular and respiratory systems may be tested. There may be significant overlap between subjects tested in 'anatomy' questions, and those tested in 'technical skills'.

1. Antecubital fossa and wrist blocks

Questions

a) Demonstrate the position of the biceps tendon on an actor. (2 marks)

b) Where would you palpate the brachial artery? (2 marks)

c) How would you block the *ulnar* nerve at the level of the elbow? (6 marks)

d) What areas of the hand does the ulnar nerve supply sensation to? (2 marks)

e) What landmarks would you use to block the *median* nerve at the wrist? (3 marks)

f) What is the test used to determine the integrity of the superficial and deep palmar arches called? (2 marks)

g) Demonstrate how you would perform this test. (3 marks)

Answers

a) Demonstrate the position of the biceps tendon on an actor. (2 marks)

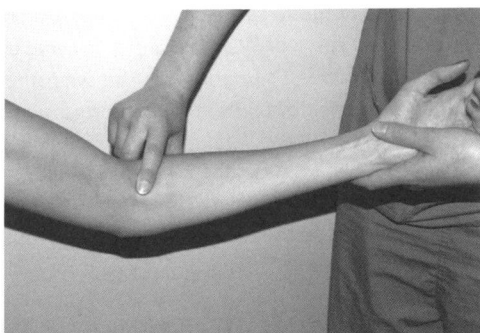

Figure 1.1 Demonstrating the position of the bicep tendon

- Flex the actor's elbow to 90°, palpating the antecubital fossa as you do so. The biceps tendon will become more prominent with elbow flexion

b) Where would you palpate the brachial artery? (2 marks)
- Anterior aspect of the antecubital fossa
- Medial to biceps tendon

c) How would you block the *ulnar* nerve at the level of the elbow? (6 marks)
- Consent, IV access, monitoring, trained assistant and resuscitation equipment
- Abduct the arm and flex to 90°
- Insert a 50mm stimulator needle 2cm proximal to ulnar sulcus
- Advance the needle at 45° cephalad to the skin
- Look for flexion of ring finger or thumb adduction
- Inject 5–10ml local anaesthetic

d) What areas of the hand does the ulnar nerve supply sensation to? (2 marks)
- Skin of the medial half of the palm and hand
- Medial $1\frac{1}{2}$ digits

e) What landmarks would you use to block the *median* nerve at the wrist? (3 marks)
- 3cm proximal to the distal palmar crease
- Between the tendons of flexor carpi radialis and palmaris longus

f) What is the test used to determine the integrity of the superficial and deep palmar arches called? (2 marks)
- Modified Allen's Test

g) Demonstrate how you would perform this test. (3 marks)
- Compress both the ulnar and radial arteries at the wrist
- Ask the patient to repeatedly clench their hand until the palm blanches
- On releasing the ulnar artery blood should return to the hand in 5–10 seconds

2. The autonomic nervous system

Questions

a) Where do the preganglionic fibres of the sympathetic nervous system originate? (2 marks)

b) Which neurotransmitter is released at sympathetic preganglionic nerve endings? (1 mark)

c) Which is the main neurotransmitter released by postganglionic sympathetic neurones? (1 mark)

d) Name two areas of the sympathetic nervous system where postganglionic fibres are exceptions to this. (3 marks)

e) Where do preganglionic fibres of the parasympathetic nervous system originate? (3 marks)

f) Name the 4 parasympathetic ganglia in the cranium. (2 marks)

g) Which neurotransmitters are released by the presynaptic and postsynaptic neurones of the parasympathetic nervous system? (2 marks)

h) What is the stellate ganglion? (2 marks)

i) Name 2 indications for a stellate ganglion block. (2 marks)

j) What features indicate that a stellate ganglion block has been successful? (2 marks)

Answers

a) Where do the preganglionic fibres of the sympathetic nervous system originate? (2 marks)
- Cell bodies in the lateral horn of (grey matter in) the spinal cord from T1 to L2

b) Which neurotransmitter is released at sympathetic preganglionic nerve endings? (1 mark)
- Acetylcholine

c) Which is the main neurotransmitter released by postganglionic sympathetic neurones? (1 mark)
- Noradrenaline

d) Name two areas of the sympathetic nervous system where postganglionic fibres are exceptions to this. (3 marks)
- Postganglionic neurones to sweat glands release acetylcholine
- Chromaffin cells of the adrenal medulla act as post ganglionic fibres and release adrenaline and noradrenaline directly into the blood

e) Where do preganglionic fibres of the parasympathetic nervous system originate? (3 marks)
- Cranial outflow from the nuclei of cranial nerves III, VII, IX and X
- Sacral outflow from S2–S4

f) Name the 4 parasympathetic ganglia in the cranium. (2 marks)
- Ciliary
- Pterygopalatine
- Otic
- Submandibular

g) Which neurotransmitters are released by the presynaptic and postsynaptic neurones of the parasympathetic nervous system? (2 marks)
- Acetylcholine is released by both pre- and postsynaptic neurones

h) What is the stellate ganglion? (2 marks)
- Sympathetic ganglion formed by the fusion of the inferior cervical and first thoracic ganglia (C7–T1)

i) Name 2 indications for a stellate ganglion block. (2 marks)
  Any 2 of:
- Vascular insufficiency: following embolectomy, Raynaud's syndrome
- Chronic pain affecting thorax or upper limb: Herpes zoster, complex regional pain syndrome, phantom limb pain, refractory angina

j) What features indicate that a stellate ganglion block has been successful? (2 marks)
- Ipsilateral Horner's Syndrome – ptosis, miosis, anhydrosis, enophthalmus

3. Base of skull

Questions

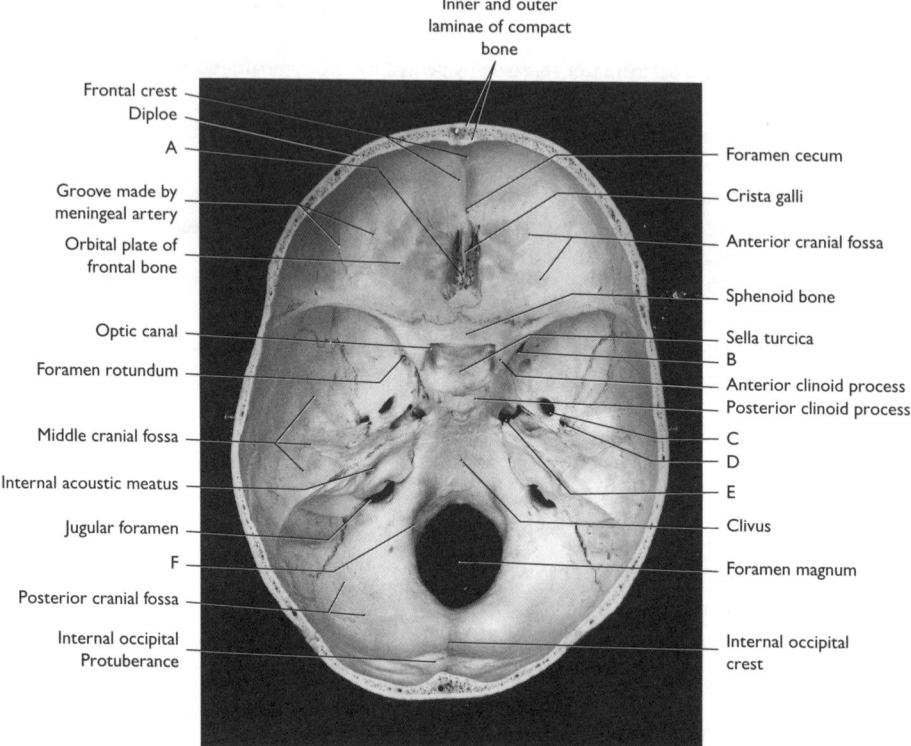

Figure 1.2 Base of Skull

Reproduced from Bruni JE and Montemurro DG, *Human Neuroanatomy: A Text, Brain Atlas, and Laboratory Dissection Guide*, copyright (2009) with permission from Oxford University USA. Adapted from Nieuwenhuys R, Voogd J, van Huijzen C. *The Human Central Nervous System. A Synopsis and Atlas*, (4th edn). Berlin: Springer–Verlag, 2008

a) Name A to F. (6 marks)

b) What structures pass through B? (3 marks)

c) What are the branches of the trigeminal nerve and what do they supply? (7 marks)

d) Through which foramen does the vagus nerve exit the skull? (1 mark)

e) Which other structures pass through this foramen? (3 marks)

Answers

a) Name A to F. (6 marks)
- A – Cribriform plate
- B – Superior orbital fissure
- C – Foramen ovale
- D – Foramen spinosum
- E – Foramen lacerum
- F – Hypoglossal canal

b) What structures pass through B? (3 marks)

Any 3 of:
- Ophthalmic division of the trigeminal nerve – CN Va (frontal, lacrimal and nasociliary branches)
- Oculomotor nerve – CN III
- Trochlear nerve – CN IV
- Abducens nerve – CN VI
- Branches of the middle meningeal and lacrimal arteries
- Sympathetic nerve fibres

c) What are the branches of the trigeminal nerve and what do they supply? (7 marks)
- Ophthalmic nerve
  - Sensory supply to the upper third of the face and frontal region of the scalp
  - Also carries sympathetic branches to the pupil (dilatation), and postganglionic parasympathetic fibres to the pupil (constriction) and lacrimal gland
- Maxillary nerve
  - Sensory supply to the middle third of the face
  - Carries postgangionic parasympathetic fibres to the lacrimal gland, sinuses, nasal, palatine and pharyngeal glands, and postganglionic taste fibres to the palatine taste buds (pregangionic fibres arise from CN VII)
- Mandibular nerve
  - Sensory supply to the lower third of the face
  - Motor supply to the muscles of mastication
  - Carries sympathetic supply and post-ganglionic parasympathetic fibres to the submandibular and sublingual glands, and postganglionic taste fibres to the anterior two thirds of the tongue (these originate from the chorda tympani branch of CN VII)

d) Through which foramen does the vagus nerve exit the skull? (1 mark)
- Jugular foramen

e) Which other structures pass through this foramen? (3 marks)
- Glossopharyngeal nerve
- Accessory nerve
- Internal jugular vein

4. Cross section of the neck at C6

Questions

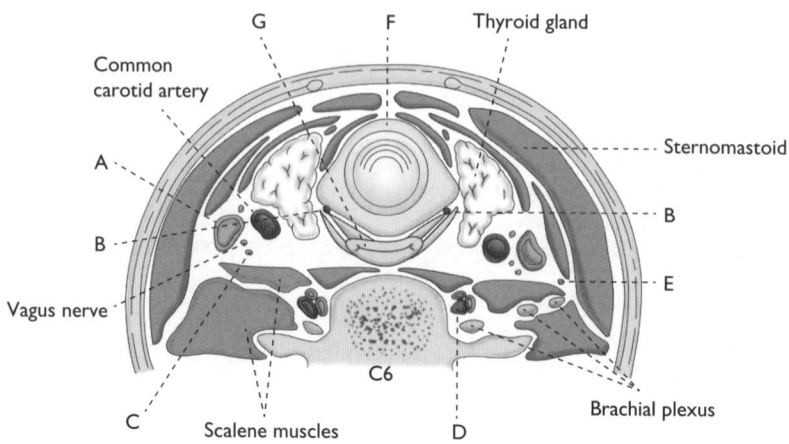

Figure 1.3 Cross section of the neck at C6

Adapted from Jackson G, et al., *Practical Procedures in Anaesthesia and Critical Care*, 2010, with permission from Oxford University Press

a) Name structure A. (1 mark)
b) Describe its course and anatomical relations as it passes from the base of skull to its termination. (4 marks)
c) What is enclosed within the carotid sheath? (3 marks)
d) Name nerve B. (1 mark)
e) Summarise the motor innervation of the larynx. (2 marks)
f) Name structure C. (1 mark)
g) Name structure D. (1 mark)
h) Describe the origin and course of this structure. (2 marks)
i) Name structure E. (1 mark)
j) From what nerve roots does structure E arise? (1 mark)
k) Name structure F. (1 mark)
l) Name structure G. (1 mark)
m) At what level in the neck does this structure originate? (1 mark)

Answers

a) Name structure A. (1 mark)
- Right internal jugular vein

b) Describe its course and anatomical relations as it passes from the base of skull to its termination. (4 marks)
- Passes through the jugular foramen
- Descends the neck in the carotid sheath adjacent to the vagus nerve
- Initially runs lateral to the internal carotid artery, and then lateral and anterior to the common carotid in the lower part of the neck
- Coalesces with the brachial vein to form the brachiocephalic vein

c) What is enclosed within the carotid sheath? (3 marks)
- Common carotid artery
- Internal jugular vein
- Vagus nerve

d) Name nerve B. (1 mark)
- Recurrent laryngeal nerve

e) Summarise the motor innervation of the larynx. (2 marks)
- Recurrent laryngeal nerve supplies all the intrinsic muscles of the larynx except cricothyroid
- Cricothyroid muscle is supplied by the external branch of the superior laryngeal nerve

f) Name structure C. (1 mark)
- Sympathetic chain

g) Name structure D. (1 mark)
- Vertebral artery

h) Describe the origin and course of this structure. (2 marks)
- Originates from the subclavian artery
- Ascends the neck anterior to the transverse processes of the cervical vertebrae

i) Name structure E. (1 mark)
- Left Phrenic nerve

j) From what nerve roots does structure E arise? (1 mark)
- C3–5

k) Name structure F. (1 mark)
- Cricoid cartilage

l) Name structure G. (1 mark)
- Oesophagus

m) At what level in the neck does this structure originate? (1 mark)
- C6

5. The diaphragm

Questions

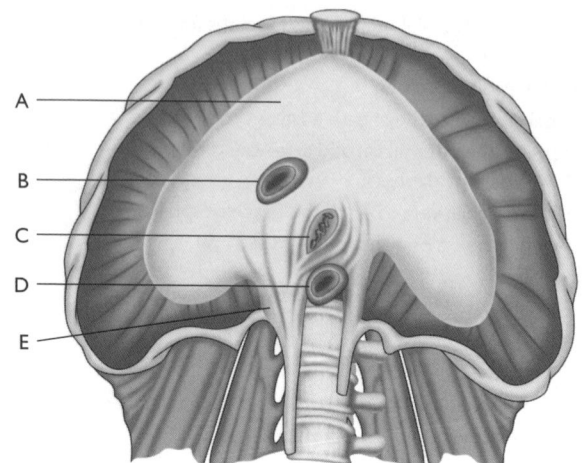

Figure 1.4 The Diaphragm

a) Name structures A, B, C, D & E. (5 marks)
b) At what level does the oesophagus pierce the diaphragm? (1 mark)
c) At what level does the aorta pierce the diaphragm? (1 mark)
d) At what level does the inferior vena cava pierce the diaphragm? (1 mark)
e) What are the attachments of the diaphragm? (6 marks)
f) What is the motor innervation of the diaphragm? (2 marks)
g) What is the sensory innervation of the diaphragm? (2 marks)
h) How would a right phrenic nerve palsy appear on a chest X-ray? (1 mark)
i) At what level does the right phrenic nerve pierce the diaphragm? (1 mark)

Answers

a) Name structures A, B, C, D & E. (5 marks)
- A – central tendon
- B – inferior vena cava
- C – oesophagus
- D – aorta
- E – right crus

b) At what level does the oesophagus pierce the diaphragm? (1 mark)
- T10

c) At what level does the aorta pierce the diaphragm? (1 mark)
- T12

d) At what level does the inferior vena cava pierce the diaphragm? (1 mark)
- T8

e) What are the attachments of the diaphragm? (6 marks)
- Anterior – lower six ribs and cartilages
- Medially – xiphisternum
- Left and right crux to lumbar vertebrae (Left L1–2, right L1–3)
- Posterior – medial arcuate ligament to psoas, lateral arcuate ligament to quadratus lumborum (2 marks)
- Centrally – pericardium

f) What is the motor innervation of the diaphragm? (2 marks)
- Phrenic nerve
- C3, 4, 5

g) What is the sensory innervation of the diaphragm? (2 marks)
- Central tendon – phrenic nerve
- Peripheries – intercostal nerves

h) How would a right phrenic nerve palsy appear on a chest X-ray? (1 mark)
- Elevation of the right hemidiaphragm

(The trachea may be deviated to the right hand side secondary to volume loss.)

i) At what level does the right phrenic nerve pierce the diaphragm? (1 mark)
- T8

6. Fetal circulation

Questions

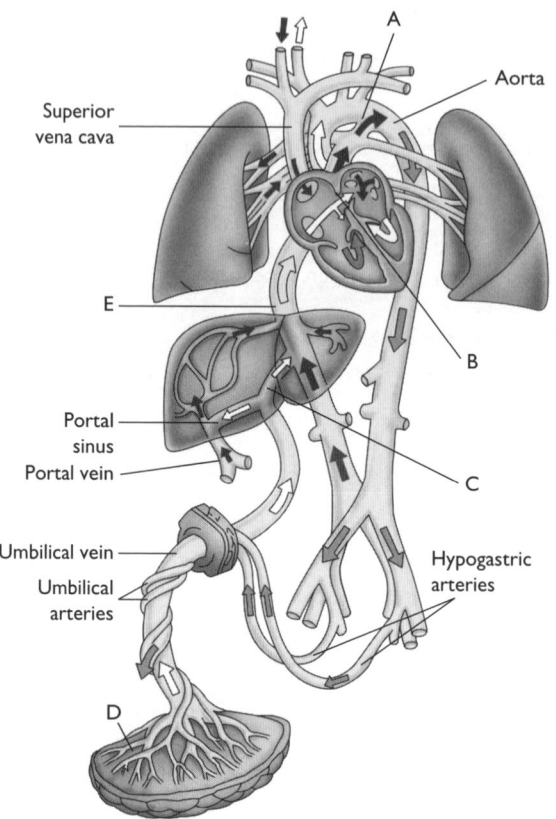

Figure 1.5 Fetal circulation
Reproduced from *Williams Obstetrics*, 23, Cunningham F, *et al.*, 90. Copyright (2010) with permission from McGraw-Hill Education

a) Name A to E. (5 marks)
b) What vessels does the umbilical cord contain? (2 marks)
c) What vessel carries oxygenated blood from the mother to the foetus? (1 mark)
d) What is the oxygen saturation of blood in the umbilical vein? (1 mark)
e) What is the oxygen saturation of blood in the foetal aorta? (1 mark)
f) When does the foramen ovale close? (1 mark)
g) By what mechanism does the foramen ovale close? (4 marks)
h) When does the ductus arteriosus usually close? (2 marks)
i) What structures does the ductus arteriosus connect? (2 marks)
j) What does the ductus arteriosus become in an adult? (1 mark)

Answers

a) Name A to E. (5 marks)
- A – Ductus arteriosus
- B – Foramen ovale
- C – Ductus venosus
- D – Placenta
- E – Inferior vena cava

b) What vessels does the umbilical cord contain? (2 marks)
- 1 umbilical vein
- 2 umbilical arteries

c) What vessel carries oxygenated blood from the mother to the foetus? (1 mark)
- Umbilical vein

d) What is the oxygen saturation of blood in the umbilical vein? (1 mark)
- 80–90%

e) What is the oxygen saturation of blood in the foetal aorta? (1 mark)
- 55%

f) When does the foramen ovale close? (1 mark)
- At birth

g) By what mechanism does the foramen ovale close? (4 marks)
- Lung expansion causes pulmonary vascular resistance to fall and pulmonary pressure to drop
- Systemic vascular resistance increases following loss of the low resistance placenta from the circulation
- Systemic pressure exceeds pulmonary pressure
- Foramen ovale flaps functionally closed

h) When does the ductus arteriosus usually close? (2 marks)
- Within 24–48hrs following birth

i) What structures does the ductus arteriosus connect? (2 marks)
- Pulmonary artery
- Descending aorta

j) What does the ductus arteriosus become in an adult? (1 mark)
- Ligamentum arteriosum

7. The heart

Questions

a) What are the layers of the heart? (3 marks)

b) Name the major coronary arteries. (3 marks)

c) Which artery supplies the SA and AV node in the majority of individuals? (2 marks)

d) Describe the venous drainage of the heart. (2 marks)

e) What is the significance of the sinus of Valsalva? (2 marks)

f) How many cusps are there in the mitral valve in the majority of individuals? (1 mark)

g) How many cusps are there in the aortic valve in the majority of individuals? (1 mark)

h) What is the normal pressure in the right atrium? (1 mark)

i) What is the normal pressure in the right ventricle? (2 marks)

j) Describe the nerve supply of the heart. (3 marks)

Answers

a) What are the layers of the heart? (3 marks)
- Endocardium
- Myocardium
- Epicardium

b) Name the major coronary arteries. (3 marks)
- Left coronary artery – divides into the circumflex artery and left anterior descending artery (anterior interventricular artery)
- Right coronary artery

c) Which artery supplies the SA and AV node in the majority of individuals? (2 marks)
- SA node right coronary (60%)
- AV node right coronary (80%)

d) Describe the venous drainage of the heart. (2 marks)
- Via the coronary sinus, which drains blood from the small, middle, oblique and great coronary veins into the right atrium
- Directly into the right atrium via anterior cardiac veins and venae chordis minimae

e) What is the significance of the sinus of Valsalva? (2 marks)
- Ensures that the leaflets of the valve do not obstruct the origins of the coronary arteries
- Functions as a blood reservoir, to allow coronary blood flow during diastole

f) How many cusps are there in the mitral valve in the majority of individuals? (1 mark)
- 2

g) How many cusps are there in the aortic valve in the majority of individuals? (1 mark)
- 3

h) What is the normal pressure in the right atrium? (1 mark)
- 0–5mmHg

i) What is the normal pressure in the right ventricle? (2 marks)
- Systolic 20–25mmHg
- Diastolic 0–5mmHg

j) Describe the nerve supply of the heart. (3 marks)
- Innervated by the cardiac plexus which contains branches from both the sympathetic and parasympathetic nervous system
- Sympathetic branches arise mainly from T1–T4 (via the cervical and upper thoracic ganglia)
- Parasympathetic branches arise from the vagus nerve

8. Anatomy of the rib

Questions

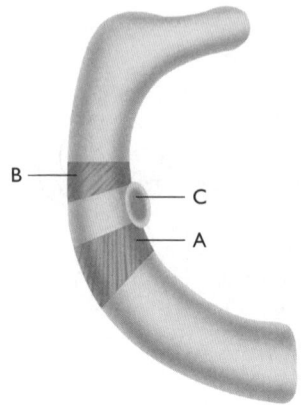

Figure 1.6 Anatomy of the rib

a) Name 3 unique features of the first rib. (3 marks)
b) What passes over structure A? (1 mark)
c) What passes over structure B? (2 marks)
d) Name structure C. (1 mark)
e) What attaches to structure C? (1 mark)
f) Regarding ribs 2–7: Which part of the rib houses the neurovascular bundle? (1 mark)
g) How are the intercostal nerve, artery and vein arranged in this groove? (3 marks)
h) Between which 2 muscular layers do the intercostal nerves run? (2 marks)
i) Name 3 indications for intercostal nerve blocks. (3 marks)
j) Where is the optimum site for performing an intercostal nerve block and why? (2 marks)
k) What is the unique feature of ribs 11 and 12? (1 mark)

Answers

a) Name 3 unique features of the first rib. (3 marks)

Any 3 of:

- Shortest
- Most curved
- There is no angle
- It has a single articular facet for articulation with the body of T1
- There are 2 grooves in the superior surface
- There is no costal groove in the inferior surface

b) What passes over structure A? (1 mark)

- Subclavian vein

c) What passes over structure B? (2 marks)

- Subclavian artery
- Lower trunk of brachial plexus

d) Name structure C. (1 mark)

- Scalene tubercle

e) What attaches to structure C? (1 mark)

- Scalenus anterior

f) Regarding ribs 2–7:

Which part of the rib houses the neurovascular bundle? (1 mark)

- The costal groove

g) How are the intercostal nerve, artery and vein arranged in this groove? (3 marks)

- Vein most superior, followed by the artery, nerve most inferior

h) Between which 2 muscular layers do the intercostal nerves run? (2 marks)

- The internal and the innermost intercostal muscles

i) Name 3 indications for intercostal nerve blocks. (3 marks)

Any 3 of:

- Rib fractures
- Thoracic surgery
- Upper abdominal surgery
- Chest drain insertion
- Breast surgery

j) Where is the optimum site for performing an intercostal nerve block and why? (2 marks)

- At the angle of the rib – to ensure that the lateral cutaneous branch is not missed
- Superior to the rib – to minimise the risk of damage to the neurovascular bundle

k) What is the unique feature of ribs 11 and 12? (1 mark)

- They are floating ribs and attach only to the vertebrae and not to the sternum

9. Spinal cord

Questions

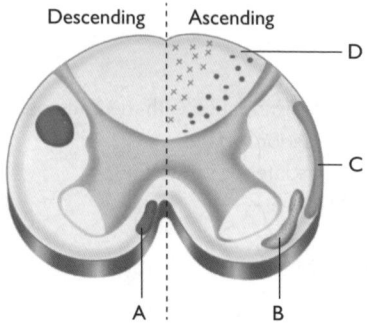

Figure 1.7 Spinal cord anatomy

a) Name A–D. (4 marks)
b) What does D transmit? (2 marks)
c) What is contained within the grey matter of the spinal cord? (2 marks)
d) Describe the blood supply to the spinal cord. (6 marks)
e) What happens if the blood flow in the anterior spinal artery ceases? (3 marks)
f) What clinical signs follow hemisection of the spinal cord? (3 marks)

Answers

a) Name A–D. (4 marks)
   - A – Anterior corticospinal tract
   - B – Spinothalamic tract
   - C – Spinocerebellar tract
   - D – Fasciculus cuneatus

b) What does D transmit? (2 marks)
   - Ipsilateral touch and proprioception
   - From the upper body

c) What is contained within the grey matter of the spinal cord? (2 marks)

   Any 2 of:
   - Neuronal cell bodies
   - Glial cells
   - Capillaries

d) Describe the blood supply to the spinal cord. (6 marks)
   - 1 anterior spinal artery
     - Originates from vertebral arteries
     - Supplies the anterior 2/3 of the spinal cord
   - 2 posterior spinal arteries
     - Originate from posterior cerebellar arteries
   - Radicular arteries from vertebral, ascending cervical, intercostal and lumbar arteries

e) What happens if the blood flow in the anterior spinal artery ceases? (3 marks)
   - Paralysis below the level of the lesion
   - Loss of pain and temperature sensation at and below the level of the lesion
   - Light touch and proprioception remain intact

f) What clinical signs follow hemisection of the spinal cord? (3 marks)
   - Ipsilateral loss of light touch and proprioception
   - Ipsilateral loss of motor function below the level of the lesion
   - Contralateral loss of pain and temperature sensation (usually 2–3 levels below the lesion)

10. Tracheobronchial tree

Questions

a) At what vertebral level does the trachea commence? (1 mark)

b) What are the anterior relations of the trachea at this level? (3 marks)

c) What are the posterior relations to the trachea at this level? (2 marks)

d) Where is a surgical tracheostomy usually inserted? (1 mark)

e) At what vertebral level does the trachea bifurcate? (1 mark)

f) What is the nerve supply to the trachea? (2 marks)

g) What are the differences between the right and left main bronchi, and what is the significance? (3 marks)

h) How many segmental bronchi are there on the right? (1 mark)

i) Name the segmental bronchi in the right upper lobe. (3 marks)

j) Which lung lobe is usually affected by aspiration? When:

   (i)   sitting (1 mark)

   (ii) lying supine (1 mark)

   (iii) lying in the left lateral position. (1 mark)

Answers

a) At what vertebral level does the trachea commence? (1 mark)
- C6

b) What are the anterior relations of the trachea at this level? (3 marks)

Any 3 of:
- Skin and subcutaneous tissue
- Strap muscles
- Isthmus of the thyroid gland
- Thyroid ima artery (where present)

c) What are the posterior relations to the trachea at this level? (2 marks)
- Oesophagus
- Recurrent laryngeal nerve (lies in the groove between the oesophagus and trachea)

d) Where is a surgical tracheostomy usually inserted? (1 mark)
- 2nd to 4th tracheal rings

e) At what vertebral level does the trachea bifurcate? (1 mark)
- T4–5

f) What is the nerve supply to the trachea? (2 marks)
- Anterior and posterior pulmonary plexuses
- Contain branches of the vagus and sympathetic nerves

g) What are the differences between the right and left main bronchi, and what is the significance? (3 marks)

Right is:
- Wider
- More vertical
- Shorter – 2.5cm versus 5cm

Foreign body is more likely to lodge in the right main bronchus than the left.

h) How many segmental bronchi are there on the right? (1 mark)
- 10 (3 in the upper lobe, 2 in the middle lobe, 5 in the lower lobe)

i) Name the segmental bronchi in the right upper lobe. (3 marks)
- Apical
- Posterior
- Anterior

j) Which lung lobe is usually affected by aspiration? When:
  (i) Sitting (1 mark)
   - Right lower lobe
  (ii) Lying supine (1 mark)
   - Right lower lobe
  (iii) Lying in the left lateral position (1 mark)
   - Lingula

Further reading

Moore K, Daley K. *Clinically Orientated Anatomy*, (4th edn). Lippincott, Williams & Wilkins, 2008
Nicholls B, Conn D, Roberts A. The Abbott pocket guide to practical peripheral nerve blockade, *Abbott Anaesthesia*. Cambridge University Press, 2010
Whitaker R, Borley NR. *Instant Anatomy*, (2nd edn). Blackwell Science, 2000
Yentis S, Hirsch N, Smith G. *Anaesthesia and Intensive Care A-Z*, (3rd edn). Elsevier, 2008

Chapter 2 **Technical Skills**

Introduction

There will be two questions on technical skills in each OSCE examination. These test practical anaesthetic skills, and background to them. You will be expected to answer questions on obtaining peripheral and central access, airway management, neuraxial blockade and peripheral nerve blocks. Even if you are unfamiliar with the procedure being examined, recalling basic concepts common to many technical skills will gain you valuable marks; for example, pre-procedure preparation (Consent, IV access, full monitoring, resuscitation equipment and trained assistance available), hand-washing and maintaining asepsis, patient positioning and aspiration prior to local anaesthetic injection.

1. Ankle block

Questions

a) Which nerve supplies the dorsum of the foot? (1 mark)

b) How would you block this nerve? (3 marks)

c) What is the cutaneous innervation of the tibial nerve? (1 mark)

d) How would you block the tibial nerve? (3 marks)

e) What cutaneous areas do the saphenous, deep peroneal and sural nerves innervate? (3 marks)

f) From which nerve does the saphenous nerve originate? (1 mark)

g) Describe the course of the saphenous nerve until the level of the ankle. (4 marks)

h) What are the maximum safe doses of bupivacaine, prilocaine and lidocaine without adrenaline? (3 marks)

i) What is the maximum safe dose of lidocaine with adrenaline? (1 mark)

Answers

a) Which nerve supplies the dorsum of the foot? (1 mark)
   - Superficial peroneal nerve
b) How would you block this nerve? (3 marks)
   - Aspirate and infiltrate subcutaneously from the lateral malleolus to the medial aspect of the tibia
   - Alternatively, infiltrate subcutaneously medially and laterally across the dorsum of the foot on a line 2–3cm distal to the inter-malleolar line
   - 10mls of local anaesthetic is a typical volume
c) What is the cutaneous innervation of the tibial nerve? (1 mark)
   - Sole of the foot (anterior and medial)
d) How would you block the tibial nerve? (3 marks)
   - Identify the midpoint of the line connecting medial malleolus and the posterior, inferior border of the calcaneum
   - Palpate the posterior tibial artery at this point
   - Insert a needle slightly lateral to the artery, and inject 5–10mls local anaesthetic as the needle is withdrawn
e) What cutaneous areas do the saphenous, deep peroneal and sural nerves innervate? (3 marks)
   - Saphenous – medial side of the ankle/foot
   - Sural – lateral side of the foot
   - Deep peroneal – web space between the first and second toes
f) From which nerve does the saphenous nerve originate? (1 mark)
   - Femoral
g) Describe the course of the saphenous nerve until the level of the ankle? (4 marks)
   - Anterior to the femoral artery within the adductor canal, until the lower edge of adductor magnus
   - Leaves adductor canal and descends along the medial side of the knee
   - Pierces the fascia lata between sartorius and gracilis and becomes subcutaneous
   - Descends behind the medial aspect of the tibia
h) What are the maximum safe doses of bupivacaine, prilocaine and lidocaine without adrenaline? (3 marks)
   - Bupivacaine – 2mg/kg
   - Prilocaine – 6mg/kg
   - Lidocaine – 3mg/kg
i) What is the maximum safe dose of lidocaine with adrenaline? (1 mark)
   - 7mg/kg

2. The brachial plexus

Questions

a) Which roots does the brachial plexus arise from? (2 marks)

b) What are formed by the combined roots? (1 mark)

c) From which roots does the middle trunk arise? (1 mark)

d) Which nerve contains branches from all of the roots? (1 mark)

e) What are the relations of the cords to the axillary artery? (3 marks)

f) From where does the lateral cutaneous nerve of the forearm arise? (1 mark)

g) Describe how you would perform an interscalene block (without ultrasound). (7 marks)

h) Name 3 complications of an interscalene block? (3 marks)

i) Which nerve is most commonly missed in an interscalene block? (1 mark)

Answers

a) Which roots does the brachial plexus arise from? (2 marks)
  - C5, C6, C7, C8, T1 – Must specify C8 for 2 marks
b) What are formed by the combined roots? (1 mark)
  - Trunks
c) From which roots does the middle trunk arise? (1 mark)
  - C7 only
d) Which nerve contains branches from all of the roots? (1 mark)
  - Radial nerve
e) What are the relations of the cords to the axillary artery? (3 marks)
  - Posterior
  - Lateral
  - Medial

  (Described in relation to the second part of the artery.)
f) From where does the lateral cutaneous nerve of the forearm arise? (1 mark)
  - Musculocutanous nerve
g) Describe how you would perform an interscalene block (without ultrasound). (7 marks)
  - Consent, monitoring, intravenous (IV) access, trained assistant, resuscitation equipment
  - Patient supine with head turned to the contralateral side
  - Palpate the interscalene groove: identify the posterior border of sternocleidomastoid at the level of the cricoid cartilage, and slide fingers laterally palpating the groove
  - Clean the skin and infiltrate local anaesthetic
  - Direct a 50mm insulated needle medially, posteriorly and caudally
  - Look for deltoid contraction or elbow flexion
  - Inject 20–40ml of local anaesthetic following negative aspiration
h) Name 3 complications of an interscalene block. (3 marks)

  Any 3 of:
  - Recurrent laryngeal nerve block
  - Horner's syndrome
  - Pneumothorax
  - Extradural or spinal block
  - Phrenic nerve block
  - Intra-arterial injection (vertebral artery)
i) Which nerve is most commonly missed in an interscalene block? (1 mark)
  - Ulnar nerve

3. Caudal epidural anaesthesia

Questions

a) List the contents of the caudal epidural space. (3 marks)

b) Describe the surface landmarks used to perform a caudal epidural injection. (3 marks)

c) Name 3 procedures for which a caudal epidural block may provide intraoperative analgesia. (3 marks)

d) Describe the Armitage regime. (4 marks)

e) Name 4 criteria to be met prior to discharge following a single shot caudal injection. (4 marks)

f) State 3 complications of caudal epidural anaesthesia. (3 marks)

Answers

a) List the contents of the caudal epidural space. (3 marks)

Any 3 of:

- Fatty and areolar connective tissue
- Venous plexus
- Sacral nerve roots
- Dural sac – terminating at the level of the second sacral vertebra

b) Describe the surface landmarks used to perform a caudal epidural injection. (3 marks)

- Injection is via the sacral hiatus
- Hiatus is bounded laterally by the 2 sacral cornua
- Supralateral elements of the posterior superior ilial spines and the apex of the sacral hiatus form an equilateral triangle

c) Name 3 procedures for which a caudal epidural block may provide intraoperative analgesia. (3 marks)

Any 3 of:

- Circumcision
- Orchidopexy
- Hydrocoele repair
- Hypospadias repair
- Inguinal hernia repair
- Umbilical hernia repair
- Lower limb procedures

d) Describe the Armitage regime. (4 marks)

- Refers to the volume of 0.25% bupivacaine required to produce a certain level of block following paediatric caudal injection
- 0.5ml/kg 0.25% bupivacaine for sacrolumbar block
- 1ml/kg upper-abdominal block
- 1.2ml/kg mid-thoracic block

e) Name 4 criteria to be met prior to discharge following a single shot caudal injection. (4 marks)

Any 4 of:

- Awake and alert with stable vital signs
- Passed urine
- Age appropriate ambulation
- Mild or absent pain
- Mild or absent postoperative nausea and vomiting (PONV)
- Written instructions for on-going care and contact details in case of problems

f) State 3 complications of caudal epidural anaesthesia. (3 marks)

Any 3 of:

- Failure or inadequate block
- Dural puncture
- Vascular puncture +/− intravascular injection
- Systemic toxicity
- Epidural abscess
- Epidural haematoma
- Urinary retention

4. Cricoid pressure and cricothyroidotomy

Questions

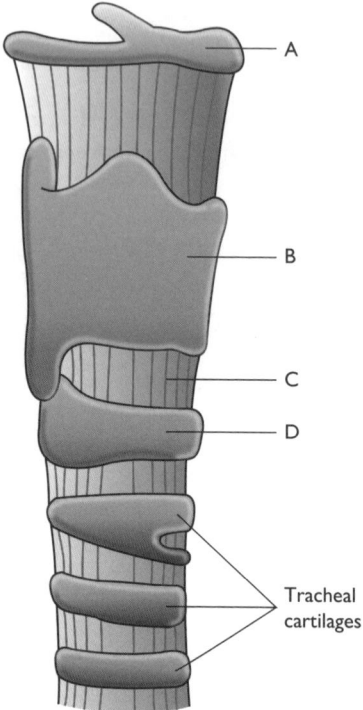

Figure 2.1 Airway Cartilage

Reproduced from Spoors, C and Kiff, K. *Training in Anaesthesia*, 2010 with permission from Oxford University Press

a) What are the indications for the use of cricoid pressure? (2 marks)
b) How much pressure should be applied during cricoid pressure for an RSI? (2 marks)
c) Explain the anatomy pertinent to cricoid pressure. (3 marks)
d) When should cricoid pressure be removed? (2 marks)
e) Look at Figure 2.1. Identify A to D. (4 marks)
f) Describe a simple technique for emergency surgical cricothyroid access. (7 marks)

Answers

a) What are the indications for the use of cricoid pressure? (2 marks)
- As part of a rapid sequence induction
- To aid visualisation of the laryngeal inlet when intubating

b) How much pressure should be applied during cricoid pressure for an RSI? (2 marks)
- 20N when awake
- 30N when anaesthetised

c) Explain the anatomy pertinent to cricoid pressure. (3 marks)
- The cricoid cartilage is a complete ring
- Backward pressure compresses the oesophagus between the posterior aspect of the cricoid cartilage and the vertebra behind
- Compression of the oesophagus prevents passive regurgitation during induction

d) When should cricoid pressure be removed? (2 marks)
- When intubation is confirmed with an appropriate end-tidal CO_2 trace
- During active vomiting

e) Look at Figure 2.1. Identify A to D. (4 marks)
- A – hyoid
- B – thyroid cartilage
- C – cricothyroid membrane
- D – cricoid cartilage

f) Describe a simple technique for emergency surgical cricothyroid access. (7 marks)

Any 7 of:
- Call for help
- If a second operator is available, then continue attempts to oxygenate from the top end
- Position the patient with the neck extended and locate the cricothyroid membrane between the thyroid and cricoid cartilages
- Using a scalpel make a long vertical incision on the neck centred on the cricothyroid membrane as identified by surface landmarks
- Secure the larynx between the thumb and the second finger
- Make a horizontal incision into the cricothyroid membrane
- Dilate the incision with either a finger or the blunt end of the scalpel
- Keeping the scalpel in the incision insert a bougie alongside into the trachea, then remove the scalpel
- Railroad an appropriately sized endotracheal or tracheostomy tube e.g. size 6 reinforced tube
- Connect to an anaesthetic circuit and confirm ventilation

5. Femoral nerve block

Questions

a) Describe how to perform a femoral nerve block. (6 marks)
b) Will a femoral nerve block alone provide effective post-operative analgesia for a knee replacement? (1 mark)
c) Which nerve supplies adductor longus? (1 mark)
d) What are the nerve roots of the obturator nerves? (2 marks)
e) What are the nerve roots of the femoral nerves? (2 marks)
f) Explain how to block the ilioinguinal nerve? (5 marks)
g) When using a peripheral nerve stimulator for regional blocks, what is the frequency of stimulus? (1 mark)
h) What is the duration of the stimulus? (1 mark)
i) Twitches at what current suggest the stimulator needle may be intraneural? (1 mark)

Answers

a) Describe how to perform a femoral nerve block. (6 marks)
- Consent, trained assistant, monitoring, IV access, resuscitation equipment
- Palpate the femoral artery at the midpoint between the superior anterior iliac spine and the pubic tubercle (= midpoint of the inguinal ligament)
- Introduce a 50mm stimulator needle LATERAL to the femoral pulse
- Look for contraction of quadriceps ('patellar dance')
- Aspirate
- Following negative aspiration inject 10–20ml of local anaesthetic

b) Will a femoral nerve block alone provide effective post-operative analgesia for a knee replacement? (1 mark)
- No. The knee joint is supplied by the sciatic and obturator nerves, in addition to the femoral nerve

c) Which nerve supplies adductor longus? (1 mark)
- Obturator nerve

d) What are the nerve roots of the obturator nerves? (2 marks)
- L2, L3, L4

e) What are the nerve roots of the femoral nerves? (2 marks)
- L2 L3, L4

f) Explain how to block the ilioinguinal nerve? (5 marks)
- Consent, trained assistant, monitoring, IV access, resuscitation equipment
- Landmark – 2cm medial to the anterior superior iliac spine
- Insert a short bevelled needle perpendicular to the skin
- Advance the needle until 2 'clicks' are felt
- Aspirate and inject 10mls of local anaesthetic

g) When using a peripheral nerve stimulator for regional blocks, what is the frequency of stimulus? (1 mark)
- 1–2Hz

h) What is the duration of the stimulus? (1 mark)
- 50–100ms

i) Twitches at what current suggest the stimulator needle may be intraneural? (1 mark)
- Less than 0.3mA

6. Intraosseous access

Questions

a) Up to what age can intraosseous (IO) access be used? (1 mark)
b) What are the landmarks for intraosseous (IO) access in the proximal tibia in adults? (2 marks)
c) Explain how to gain intraosseous access. (8 marks)
d) What are the relative contraindications for intraosseous access insertion? (3 marks)
e) What are the complications? (3 marks)
f) What volume of fluid bolus should be used to resuscitate a 4-year-old boy? (3 marks)

Answers

a) Up to what age can IO access be used? (1 mark)
- There is no age limit (intraosseous access is now recommended for both paediatric and adult life support)

b) What are the landmarks for IO access in the proximal tibia in adults? (2 marks)
- Anterior surface
- 2–3cm below the tibial tuberosity

c) Explain how to gain intraosseous access. (8 marks)
- Stabilise the limb on a firm surface
- Identify the landmarks and clean the skin
- Check the patency of the cannula and flush attachments
- Insert the needle at 90 degrees to the skin
- Advance the needle until a give is felt, and the needle remains stable in an upright position
- Remove the trochar, attach a syringe and ensure bone marrow can be aspirated
- Check the cannula flushes easily with saline and there is no extravasation
- Secure

d) What are the relative contraindications for intraosseous access insertion? (3 marks)
Any 3 of:
- Fractured bone or fracture proximal to IO insertion point
- Loss of skin integrity or infection
- Osteogenesis imperfecta
- Osteoporosis
- Coagulopathy

e) What are the complications? (3 marks)
Any 3 of:
- Infection
- Compartment syndrome
- Fracture
- Extravasation
- Embolism

f) What volume of fluid bolus should be used to resuscitate a 4-year-old boy? (3 marks)
- Weight = (age + 4) × 2
  = (4 + 4) × 2 = 16kg
- Fluid bolus = 20ml/kg = 20 × 16 = 320ml

7. Laryngeal mask airway (LMA) insertion

Questions

a) Name 4 advantages of the laryngeal mask airway (LMA) over the endotracheal tube. (4 marks)

b) Describe how you would prepare and insert a classic LMA. (5 marks)

c) Where is the tip of the LMA located once correctly positioned? (1 mark)

d) What size LMA would you use for a 19kg child? (1 mark)

e) What is the maximum volume of air that should be inserted into this LMA? (1 mark)

f) What is the maximum recommended cuff pressure? (1 mark)

g) What steps may be taken to improve the seal if the oropharyngeal leak pressure is low on hand ventilation? (3 marks)

h) Name 2 complications associated with the use of a LMA. (2 marks)

i) What are the 2 major advantages of a LMA Proseal™? (2 marks)

Answers

a) Name 4 advantages of the laryngeal mask airway (LMA) over the endotracheal tube. (4 marks)

Any 4 of:

- Speed of placement
- Ease of placement
- Haemodynamic stability on insertion
- Lower incidence of sore throat
- Reduced anaesthetic requirement to facilitate insertion
- Reduced anaesthetic requirement for airway tolerance
- Minimal increase in intraocular pressure on insertion
- Lower incidence of coughing during emergence

b) Describe how you would prepare and insert a classic LMA. (5 marks)

- Inflate the cuff to check patency and then deflate
- Lubricate the posterior aspect of the cuff
- Hold between the thumb and the index finger and use the index finger to guide the airway along the hard palate until resistance is met
- Insert an appropriate volume of air into the cuff and allow the LMA to rise out of the mouth (up to 20ml for size 3, 30ml for a size 4, 40ml for size 5)
- Connect to an anaesthetic circuit and, if necessary, insert more air (up to the recommended maximum) into the cuff to eliminate leak

c) Where is the tip of the LMA located once correctly positioned? (1 mark)

- At the top of the oesophagus

d) What size LMA would you use for a 19kg child? (1 mark)

- Size 2

e) What is the maximum volume of air that should be inserted into this LMA? (1 mark)

- 10mls

f) What is the maximum recommended cuff pressure? (1 mark)

- $60cmH_2O$

g) What steps may be taken to improve the seal if the oropharyngeal leak pressure is low on hand ventilation? (3 marks)

- Inject further air into the cuff not exceeding the maximum volume or pressure
- Adjust the position of the LMA
- Replace the LMA with the next size up

h) Name 2 complications associated with the use of a LMA. (2 marks)

Any 2 of:

- Sore throat
- Aspiration of gastric contents
- Airway obstruction due to folding over of the cuff tip

i) What are the 2 major advantages of a LMA Proseal™? (2 marks)

- Higher oropharyngeal leak pressures
- Gastric drainage port

8. Anatomy of the orbit and peribulbar anaesthesia

Questions

a) Name the branches of the ophthalmic nerve supplying sensation to the globe. (2 marks)
b) Summarise the motor innervation of the extra-ocular muscles. (3 marks)
c) Name 4 structures transmitted through the superior orbital fissure. (4 marks)
d) Describe an approach to performing a peribulbar block. (6 marks)
e) What type and volume of local anaesthetic will you use? (1 mark)
f) Name 3 complications of this procedure. (3 marks)

Answers

a) Name the branches of the ophthalmic nerve supplying sensation to the globe. (2 marks)
- Long and short posterior ciliary nerves

b) Summarise the motor innervation of the extra-ocular muscles. (3 marks)
- Oculomotor nerve (CN III) supplies superior, inferior and medial recti
- Abducens nerve (CN VI) supplies lateral rectus
- Trochlear nerve (CN IV) supplies superior oblique

c) Name 4 structures transmitted through the superior orbital fissure. (4 marks)
Any 4 of:
- Lacrimal nerve
- Trochlear nerve
- Nasociliary nerve
- Frontal nerve
- Abducens nerve
- Oculomotor nerve
- Superior ophthalmic vein

(Mnemonic: Late trainees never fail to annoy old surgeons.)

d) Describe an approach to performing a peribulbar block. (6 marks)
(NB. One and two injection techniques have been described.)
- Apply topical anaesthesia and ask the patient to look straight ahead
- Inferolateral injection: A 25mm 25G needle is inserted through the lower lid, at the junction between the lateral third and medial two thirds
    - Needle is directed backwards and inferiorly to contact bone, and then redirected posteriorly under the globe to approximately 20–25mm
- Second injection using 25mm 25G needle
    - Either superiorly, through the upper lid, at the junction between the medial third and lateral two thirds of the edge of the roof of the orbit
    - Or insert medial to the medial caruncle – initially direct backwards and medially to hit the orbit wall, then redirect parallel to the medial wall
- Local anaesthetic should only be injected following negative aspiration
- Apply light pressure to the eye using a soft pad or a Honan's balloon

e) What type and volume of local anaesthetic will you use? (1 mark)
- Total of 5 to 10mls (usually 4–6ml for the inferolateral injection and 3–5ml for the second injection)

(Because peribulbar blocks are extraconal, the volume of local must be greater than for retrobulbar blocks, to allow spread into the intraconal space, where the nerves to be blocked are located.)

f) Name 3 complications of this procedure. (3 marks)
Any 3 of:
- Globe perforation
- Retrobulbar haematoma formation (less likely if a needle less than 31mm is used)
- Spinal anaesthesia
- Optic nerve trauma

9. Spinal anaesthesia

Questions

a) What anatomical landmarks does Tuffier's line correspond to? (2 marks)

b) At what level does the spinal cord end in adults? (1 mark)

c) How do you position a patient for spinal anaesthesia in the lateral position? (3 marks)

d) Explain your approach to performing a spinal anaesthetic for elective knee surgery. (8 marks)

e) What are the absolute contraindications to spinal anaesthesia? (3 marks)

f) What is the total volume of cerebrospinal fluid (CSF) in an adult? (1 mark)

g) What is the specific gravity of CSF? (1 mark)

h) What is the specific gravity of heavy bupivacaine? (1 mark)

Answers

a) What anatomical landmarks does Tuffier's line correspond to? (2 marks)
   - Iliac crests
   - L4 vertebra

b) At what level does the spinal cord end in adults? (1 mark)
   - L1–2

c) How do you position a patient for spinal anaesthesia in the lateral position? (3 marks)
   - Back flexed and close to the edge of the table or bed
   - Chin on chest
   - Knees drawn up towards the chest

d) Explain your approach to performing a spinal anaesthetic for elective knee surgery (8 marks)
   - Consent, full monitoring, resuscitation equipment and trained assistant
   - Large bore IV access with fluids connected
   - Asepsis – hat, gloves, gown and mask for operator; chlorhexidine to the patient's skin
   - Identify landmarks and aim for L3/4, L4/5 or L5/S1 interspaces. Apply local anaesthesia to the skin
   - Insert the spinal needle in the midline, and advance until a 'dural click' is felt
   - With one hand steadying the bevel, use the other hand to remove the stylet and confirm free flow of cerebral spinal fluid (CSF)
   - Attach the syringe of appropriate local anaesthetic +/− opioid, aspirate CSF and inject slowly, aspirate again at the end of injection
   - Remove the needle, and cover the injection site

e) What are the absolute contraindications to spinal anaesthesia? (3 marks)
   - Anticoagulation or coagulation abnormalities
   - Localised infection overlying insertion site
   - Patient refusal

f) What is the total volume of CSF in an adult? (1 mark)
   - 100–150ml

g) What is the specific gravity of CSF? (1 mark)
   - 1.006–1.009

h) What is the specific gravity of heavy bupivacaine? (1 mark)
   - 1.026

10. Subclavian central venous line insertion

Questions

a) Which routes can be used for central venous line insertion? (3 marks)

b) What are the benefits of using the subclavian route? (3 marks)

c) Name 2 absolute contraindications to subclavian line insertion? (2 marks)

d) Explain how you would insert a subclavian central venous line. (8 marks)

e) What would you do following completion of the procedure? (2 marks)

f) Name the 2 main complications of subclavian line insertion. (2 marks)

Answers

a) Which routes can be used for central venous line insertion? (3 marks)
- Internal jugular vein
- Femoral vein
- Subclavian vein

b) What are the benefits of using the subclavian route? (3 marks)
- Lower infection risk than other routes
- Increased comfort for the patient
- Can be used in patients with suspected cervical spine injury

c) Name 2 absolute contraindications to subclavian line insertion? (2 marks)
- Patient refusal
- Coagulopathy

d) Explain how you would insert a subclavian central venous line. (8 marks)
- Position the patient – supine, head down
- Wash hands and use aseptic technique – hat, gloves, gown, mask, 2% chlorhexidine to the skin, drape
- Identify the landmarks – 1cm below the clavicle at the junction between the middle and the medial thirds
- Direct the needle towards the suprasternal notch, while continuously aspirating on the syringe
- Confirm that the blood is venous by transducing or performing a blood gas
- Continue to insert the line using a Seldinger technique
- Ensure all lumens aspirate and flush easily
- Secure and apply a transparent dressing

e) What would you do following completion of the procedure? (2 marks)
- Chest X-ray (even if the procedure is unsuccessful)
- Document the procedure in the notes

f) Name the 2 main complications of subclavian line insertion. (2 marks)
- Pneumothorax
- Arterial puncture (and possible haemothorax)

Further reading

Difficult Airway Society, Failed Ventilation (2007). Available at: http://www.das.uk.com/guidelines/cvci.html
Gabbott D. Recent advances in airway technology. *Contin Educ Anaesth Crit Care Pain*, 1 (3): 76–80, 2001
Jackson G, Soni N, Whiten C. *Practical procedures in anaesthesia and critical care*. Oxford University Press, 2011
New York School of Regional Anaesthesia, Local and regional anaesthesia for eye surgery. Available at: http://www.nysora.com/mobile/regional-anesthesia/sub-specialties/3029-local-regional-anesthesia-for-eye-surgery.html
Nicholls B, Conn D, Roberts A. The Abbott pocket guide to practical peripheral nerve blockade. *Abbott Anaesthesia*, 2010

Chapter 3 **History**

Introduction

There are two history stations in the OSCE. Marks are awarded for quickly and concisely obtaining the information necessary to conduct safe anaesthesia. It is important to demonstrate knowledge of a topic by asking the right questions and therefore it is also important to practice this skill before the exam.

One approach is to get all the essential information out of the way in the first few minutes; for example, a brief past medical history, drug history, anaesthetic history, allergies, fasting status, smoking and alcohol history and exercise tolerance. You can then take your time to explore whatever comes up in this brief overview.

It is essential to cover all the components of the history even if only briefly. Try to develop your own battery of questions to get through the essential information in a quick, stylish manner.

In the following examples, a full history has not been elicited every time to allow practice in different areas and avoid repetition of the same questions. Try adding your set of questions at the start or end of these scenarios to make sure all the history is covered.

All history stations should be started with you introducing yourself, confirming the patient's identity and confirming what operation is being discussed.

1. Patient with previous intensive care admission

Questions

Please take an anaesthetic history from this 45-year-old man, presenting for a knee arthroscopy, who previously had a splenectomy and has been in intensive care following a road traffic accident.

a) How do you want to start the interview and what do you want to know about the operation? (5 marks)
b) What further information do you need with regard to the splenectomy? (6 marks)
c) What do you want to know about his intensive care admission? (9 marks)

Answers

a) How do you want to start the interview and what do you want to know about the operation? (5 marks)
- Firstly, start by introducing yourself, confirming the patient's full name and age / date of birth
- Confirm which knee he is expecting to have the operation on
- You must ask why he is having the knee arthroscopy and if it is associated with any other diseases
- Explore any associated diseases. Common orthopaedic operations are associated with rheumatological disease. This has a number of implications:
  - Airway management may be difficult due to atlanto-axial instability, cricoarytenoid involvement or restricted movement of the neck or jaw. A full airway assessment is required in these cases
  - Systemic manifestations of rheumatological disease may affect perioperative care e.g. lung, cardiac or renal complications of rheumatoid disease
  - Patients may be taking a range of immunosuppressive, analgesic or disease modifying medications to control their disease. These have a range of side effects and further investigations may need to be performed
  - Regional anaesthesia may be more difficult in patients with fixed deformities or contractures
  - Positioning of patients on the operating table may be more difficult and they may be at increased risk of compression neuropathy

b) What further information do you need with regard to the splenectomy? (6 marks)
- Confirm why and when the splenectomy was performed
  - Indications for splenectomy:
    - Idiopathic thrombocytopaenic purpura
    - Traumatic rupture or haemorrhage
    - Tumour
    - Splenomegaly secondary to infection
    - Functional asplenia also may occur with conditions such as sickle cell disease and similar precautions should be taken
- Ask him what vaccinations he received around the time of the splenectomy, and when he last had any boosters
  - Asplenic patients are at risk of overwhelming post-splenectomy infection (OPSI) when exposed to encapsulated organisms
  - Two weeks after emergency splenectomy patients should be immunized to cover *Pneumococcus, Haemophilus influenzae* and *Neisseria meningitidis*. They should receive annual influenza immunizations and 5-yearly pneumococcal vaccine boosters
- Check that he is prescribed regular prophylactic antibiotics post splenectomy and has been compliant with this medication

Asplenic patients must receive at least two years of prophylactic antibiotics. The majority will take Penicillin V (Clarithromycin if penicillin allergic). Life-long prophylaxis is recommended but non-compliance is common. Life-long antibiotics are essential in patients at high risk of pneumococcal infection e.g. those younger than 16 or older than 50 years of age and those who have had a previous invasive pneumococcal infection or a poor serological response to immunization.

c) What do you want to know about his intensive care admission? (9 marks)

- What other injuries did he sustain?
  - Long term complications of injuries sustained in the past may influence choice of anaesthesia and perioperative care e.g. intra-cranial insult, spinal injury, thoracic injury or gastrointestinal trauma
- Did he require prolonged ventilatory support? If so, did he require a tracheostomy?
- Tracheostomy following a road traffic accident could be performed for a number of reasons:
  - Prolonged ventilatory wean due to recurrent infection or muscle weakness
  - Trauma to the neck and/or upper airway
  - Failed extubation due to slow neurological recovery
  - It is important to establish the reason for tracheostomy, the amount of time it was in situ and how recently a normal airway was re-established as these factors may influence the anatomy of the airway and ease of intubation
- Has he had any problems with breathing or voice changes since? Has he been reviewed by an ear, nose and throat (ENT) surgeon, or had any scans of his neck?
  - Long term complications of tracheostomy include:
    - Tracheal stenosis
    - Tracheomalacia
    - Tracheosophageal fistula
    - Vocal cord oedema or distortion

Certain symptoms may indicate tracheal pathology such as voice change, hoarseness and difficulty in breathing on exertion. Such patients should have been investigated with a computerised axial tomography scan (CT) of their neck to assess tracheal calibre, and nasoendoscopy, bronchoscopy or pulmonary function tests to investigate dynamic obstruction. However, recent studies have shown that nearly half of patients with moderate stenosis post-tracheostomy are asymptomatic. Elucidating whether the patient has been intubated at any point since the tracheostomy was removed may also be helpful.

2. The adult diabetic patient

Questions

Please take an anaesthetic history from this 38-year-old woman presenting for a manipulation under anaesthesia (MUA) of her wrist following a fall. She has diabetes.

a) How would you begin the interview and what would you want to know about the fall? (4 marks)
b) What do you what to ask first about her diabetes? (2 marks)
c) How might you assess the severity of her diabetes in the history? (6 marks)
d) How else might you assess how well her diabetes is controlled? (3 marks)
e) What other past medical history is it important to ask about? (2 marks)
f) What do you want to know about her drug history? (3 marks)

DM — T1 /T2 .

— Current treatment + 1°/2° prevention

⇒ complication —> micro —> renal /eye disease /neuropathy

—> macro —> MI/stroke

—> HbA1c / glucose measurements @ home

—> Co-morbidities

∟ ↑ BP

∟ ↑ cholesterol

Answers

a) How would you begin the interview and what would you want to know about the fall? (4 marks)
- Firstly, start by introducing yourself, confirming the patient's full name and age / date of birth
- Confirm which wrist she is expecting to have surgery on
- What was the mechanism of injury?
- Make sure that this was a truly mechanical fall and wasn't associated with an undiagnosed infection, syncope or arrhythmia
- Did she sustain any other injuries?
  - All trauma patients should be assessed for signs and symptoms of other traumatic injuries. The mechanism of injury can indicate the likelihood of significant thoracic, abdominal, head or long bone injuries. It is important to make sure that they have been investigated, and to take into account the implications of, for example, an untreated pneumothorax or intracranial haemorrhage for their perioperative care

b) What do you what to ask first about her diabetes? (2 marks)
- When was it diagnosed?
  - The duration of disease is important in diabetes as increasing duration is associated with an increased risk of micro- and macrovascular complications. Other risk factors for complications in diabetes include:
    - Poor blood sugar control
    - Obesity
    - Hypertension
    - Hyperlipidaemia
    - Smoking
- Does she have type 1 or type 2 diabetes?
  - This has implications about what associated morbidity she may have and what treatment regimens she maybe on

c) How might you assess the severity of her diabetes in the history? (6 marks)
- You need to ask about the complications of diabetes
  - Microvascular – has she ever seen a kidney doctor? Is she up-to-date with retinal screening? What did it show? Has she lost feeling in her feet or fingertips? Does she suffer from reflux or constipation?
  - Macrovascular – has she ever had a MI or stroke?

d) How else might you assess how well her diabetes is controlled? (3 marks)
- Ask if she regularly checks her blood sugars
- If so, what have they been over the last few days and this morning?
- Does she know her latest glycated haemoglobin (HbA1c) level?
  - It is important to assess the patient's recent and longer-term blood sugar control. This is a trauma patient who may have been starved for several procedures or not been able to use their 'usual' insulin regimen. Maintaining blood sugars between 6–10mmol/l has been shown to improve perioperative outcomes. HaemoglobinA1c is a marker of medium term control and a level >8% is associated with adverse perioperative outcomes; in the elective setting it might be appropriate to postpone such patients and liaise with their general practitioner (GP) about optimizing the control

e) What other past medical history is it important to ask about? (2 marks)
- Does she suffer from hypertension or high cholesterol?
  - ♦ Co-morbidities are common associations with both types of diabetes and should be explored even in younger patients. They also increase the risk of diabetic complications

f) What do you want to know about her drug history? (3 marks)
- What insulin regimen does she use? What has she taken in the last 24 hours?
- How did she use her insulin in view of the need to starve for 6 hours?
- Does she take any oral hypoglycaemics? Has she continued to take these in the last 24 hours?
  - ♦ Patients with type 1 diabetes may be on a range of medications:
    - Rapidly acting insulins include: insulin aspart, insulin lispro
    - Long acting insulins include: glargine, detemir
    - Patients are commonly on a basal/bolus regimen, which includes both. It is important to establish when they have used insulin in the past 24 hours and if they have adjusted their dosing to account for a period of starvation. Patients are now presenting with ambulatory continuous infusion pumps and their usual insulin intake should be calculated. Oral hypoglycaemics are important as the patient may have continued taking them despite fasting. Metformin can cause lactic acidosis perioperatively

Further information about the complications of diabetes and their importance in the perioperative period:
- Microvascular complications:
  - ♦ Nephropathy – the patient may be anywhere on the spectrum from having subclinical renal impairment to having had a renal transplant This has implications for the choice of drugs and post-operative management
  - ♦ Retinopathy – there is a strong association between retinopathy and nephropathy in diabetics. Different forms of communication may be required for a visually-impaired patient
  - ♦ Neuropathy
    - Peripheral neuropathy. It is important to assess the neurological deficit especially if regional anaesthesia is being considered. There is no evidence that regional anaesthesia is associated with lower mortality or morbididty than general anaesthesia
    - Autonomic neuropathy is present in 50% of patients with type 1 diabetes. Gastroparesis is common and puts the patient at greater risk of aspiration and post-operative nausea and vomiting. Cardiac dysfunction may be highlighted by postural hypotension or lack of heart rate variability and indicates severe autonomic dysfunction. This puts the patient at risk of arrhythmias and labile blood pressure perioperatively
- Macrovascular complications:
  - ♦ Although more common with type 2 diabetes, type 1 diabetes patients are at risk of ischaemic heart disease and cerebrovascular disease especially if co-morbidities such as hypertension, hyperlipidaemia and nephropathy are present
- Other complications:
  - ♦ Type 1 diabetes is associated with 'stiff joint syndrome' which can affect jaw opening

3. Eye surgery in a patient with a cardiac history

Questions

Please take an anaesthetic history from this 78-year-old man presenting for a cataract operation. He is known to have cardiac problems.

a) How would you start the interview and what would you want to know about his ophthalmic history? (4 marks)
b) The patient tells you that he has had a heart attack in the past. What do you want to know about the myocardial infarction? (3 marks)
c) How would you assess his current cardiac function and why is this important in ophthalmic surgery? (5 marks)
d) He explains that he has been diagnosed with atrial fibrillation following the MI. What information do you want to know? (2 marks)
e) What is of particular importance in his drug history? (4 marks)
f) What else would you want to ask about in his past medical history? (2 marks)

MI - When
  - Rx → stent / CABG / medical Rx
       → antiplatelets / anti coag
    → Current therapy
    → ET → ? chest pain
    → Complication → CCF / arrhythmia .
               → ? able to lie flat

Co-morbidities
  - DM → stauratin
  - ↑BP - ↑ risk bleeding

Answers

a) How would you start the interview and what would you want to know about his ophthalmic history? (4 marks)

- Firstly, start by introducing yourself, confirming the patient's full name and age / date of birth
- Confirm which eye he is expecting to have surgery on. This is particularly important in cataract surgery as both sides are often affected but it is usual to operate on one at a time
- Determine whether he has any other eye conditions that may affect the type of anaesthesia you can offer
  - Some ophthalmic pathology, such as a previous surgery for retinal detachment, means that regional anaesthesia is contra-indicated or is much higher risk, as with raised intra-ocular pressure
- If they have had previous ophthalmic surgery, ask what type of anaesthesia they had and how the experience was

b) The patient tells you that he has had a heart attack in the past. What do you want to know about the myocardial infarction? (3 marks)

- Ask the patient how long ago the myocardial infarction (MI) was
- What treatment did he have at the time?
- Ask explicitly if he has any cardiac stents
  - Despite cataract removal being a relatively minor operation, it is recommended that it should not be done within three months of an acute coronary event. Elucidating whether the patient had conservative management, angioplasty, coronary stenting or surgery will have implications on what medication they take, and their continued risk of ischaemic events. Knowing the timing of any coronary stenting will also help when weighing up the risks and benefits of stopping anti-platelet therapy

c) How would you assess his current cardiac function and why is this important in ophthalmic surgery? (5 marks)

- Run through cardiac symptoms in a structured way – this must include asking about orthopnoea, dyspnoea, chest pain, palpitations, syncopal episodes and ankle swelling
- Ask about his exercise tolerance
- Ask the patient if he will be able to tolerate lying flat for a prolonged period of time
  - Cataract surgery is usually performed under regional anaesthesia. However, the experience can be stressful and claustrophobic for patients, potentially increasing their myocardial oxygen demand. It is therefore important to quantify their current ischaemic symptoms and any evidence of cardiac failure, valvular pathology and uncontrolled arrhythmias. Patients are required to lie flat for the operation and severe orthopnoea may prevent this. Sedation or conversion to a general anaesthetic is always a possibility so thorough pre-assessment is always required

d) He explains that he has been diagnosed with atrial fibrillation following the MI. What information do you want to know? (2 marks)

- Has he ever had a direct current (DC) cardioversion?
- Does he feel like he has on-going palpitations or 'funny heart rhythms'?
  - It is important to assess whether the patient has paroxysmal atrial fibrillation (AF) requiring cardioversion, or stable, persistent rate-controlled AF. It may also be useful to know if the patient has had any cerebrovascular events as a result of the arrhythmia as this will change the risk:benefit ratio of stopping anticoagulants / anti-platelet agents

e) What is of particular importance in his drug history? (4 marks)
- Does he take warfarin?
- Does he take antiplatelet medication?
- Explore if and when these medications were stopped?
- Has he had a recent international normalized ratio (INR) check?
  - For isolated cataract surgery it is now thought that any risks of stopping anti-platelet and anticoagulant therapy outweighs the benefit and small risk of perioperative bleeding. However, surgery should be postponed if the INR is severely deranged. This may also affect the choice of anaesthesia; for example, a patient on warfarin should not have a peribulbar block but could have a sub-Tenon's block as long as the INR was not grossly elevated

f) What else would you want to ask about in his past medical history? (2 marks)
- Hypertension
- Diabetes
- Respiratory disease
- Neurological disease
  - Poorly controlled hypertension increases the risk of bleeding and perioperative cardiovascular morbidity. Patients will still be starved for ophthalmic surgery so it is important to know if the patient has diabetes. Neurological diseases such as Parkinson's disease may rule out regional anaesthesia and severe respiratory disease may mean that the patient is unable to tolerate lying flat

4. Patient with obstructive sleep apnoea

Questions

Please take an anaesthetic history from this 48-year-old man listed for sinus surgery (a FESS procedure). He claims he is having the surgery as his wife complains that he snores heavily.

a) What would you want to know about his snoring? (2 marks)
b) What symptoms suggestive of Obstructive Sleep Apnoea (OSA) do you need to ask him about? Can you assess if he is at high risk of having OSA? (8 marks)
c) What other symptoms do you need to ask about? (4 marks)
d) What do you want to know about how he manages his OSA? (3 marks)
e) This is an ear, nose and throat (ENT) operation, what else do you need to ask about? (1 mark)
f) What else is important to know about given that he is due to have sinus surgery and the surgeons may want a bloodless field? (2 marks)

[Handwritten notes:]

OSA → snoring y/n
  → daytime tiredness
  → apnoea
  → collar size

S noring
T iredness
O bserved apnoea
P ↑BP

BMI >35
A >50 yrs
N eck circumference
Gender M >F

≥3 = ↑ risk

Related resp complication
CCF symptoms
Arrhythmias

CPAP → compliance
  → how long for
  → brought in?

Recent infection in airway (for all ENT / airway surgery)

ENT → ↓BP surgery
  Hx of stroke/TIA
  antihypertensives?

Answers

a) What would you want to know about his snoring? (2 marks)
- Has he had a formal sleep study?
- Has he had a diagnosis of OSA?
  - ♦ Formal sleep testing involves polysomnography and it is important to look at these results to assess the severity of a patient's OSA. An apnoea/hypopnea index (AHI) of ≥5/hour indicates the presence of OSA whereas an AHI of ≥30/hour is suggestive of severe OSA

b) What symptoms suggestive of OSA do you need to ask his about? Can you assess if he is at high risk of having OSA? (8 marks)
- Is he tired during the day?
- Does his wife say that he stops breathing at night?
- What is his collar size?
- What is his 'STOP BANG' score?
  - ♦ Obstructive sleep apnoea should be suspected in patients who have sleep disturbances and associated physiological risk factors. An easy screening method is the 'STOP BANG' questionnaire; patients score 1 point for each positive risk factor. The acronym stands for: S – snoring, T – tiredness during the day, O – observed cessation of breathing, P – high blood Pressure, B – BMI >35, A – Age >50 years old, N – neck circumference >40cm, G – gender (male). A score of greater than 3 is highly suggestive of OSA

c) What other symptoms do you need to ask about? (4 marks)
- Dyspnoea
- Ankle swelling
- Palpitations
- Chest pain
  - ♦ Any evidence of congestive cardiac failure or hypercarbia ($paCO_2$>6.5kPa) secondary to OSA puts the patient at higher risk of perioperative morbidity. It is suggested therefore that surgery be postponed until their condition has been optimized with lifestyle modification or nocturnal continuous positive airway pressure (CPAP). Having OSA increases cardiovascular morbidity, independent of the body mass index (BMI) of the patient. This is thought to be due to chronically elevated catecholamine levels

d) What do you want to know about how he manages his OSA? (3 marks)
- Does he use CPAP at night?
- If so, for how long has he used it?
- Does he have it with him today?
- Does he actually use it as prescribed?
  - ♦ Patients may be established on CPAP, following assessment by sleep physicians. It is important to elucidate whether they are compliant and if it has improved their symptoms. Patients should have been advised to bring their CPAP machines with them for postoperative use in recovery and on the ward. Anaesthetic agents and opiates further suppress the respiratory drive so it is crucial for patients to be monitored closely, ideally in an HDU environment

e) This is an ENT operation, what else do you need to ask about? (1 mark)
- Is the patient well today? Is there any evidence of a respiratory tract infection?
  - ♦ Any pre-operative assessment for ENT patients should include questions about active airway infection. This may lead to increased airway reactivity and an increased risk of post-operative bleeding

f) What else is important to know about given that he is due to have sinus surgery and the surgeons may want a bloodless field? (2 marks)

- Has the patient ever had a stroke or transient ischaemic attack (TIA)?
  - Is he on any antihypertensive medication?
    - During a FESS procedure, hypotensive anaesthesia may be requested by the surgical team to improve the surgical field. If the patient is hypertensive it is important to know their usual blood pressure in order to maintain cerebral perfusion. Patients with a history of TIAs or ischaemic strokes may not be suitable for induced hypotension

5. Caesarean section in a patient with ankylosing spondylitis

Questions

Please take an anaesthetic history from this 30-year-old woman who needs a category 2 Caesarean section. She is known to have ankylosing spondylitis and the foetus has intra-uterine growth retardation (IUGR).

a) What do you need to ask any woman going for Caesarean section? (7 marks)
b) She explains that she was diagnosed with ankylosing spondylitis two years ago. What do you want to know now? (3 marks)
c) What do you want to know about her treatment? (3 marks)
d) She tells you that, after a previous operation, the anaesthetist told her that it was difficult for them to put a tube in her mouth and that she should always tell anaesthetists this in the future. What should you ask? (5 marks)
e) What do you want to ask about, given that her baby has IUGR? (2 marks)

C-section   ? prev deliveries -
→ G? P?   prev problems
→ Pregnancy - GDM / ↑BP.
→ prev anaesthetic / regional / GA
→ eat / drink
→ allergies
→ PMHx

Ank spond ──→ affects spine / jaw
        └→ extra articular ──→ conduction / MV / fibrosis
                              works
        └→ Rx

Answers

a) What do you need to ask any woman going for Caesarean section? (7 marks)

- Has she had any problems in this pregnancy?
- Does she have any medical problems?
- Does she take any medication?
- Is she allergic to anything?
- Has she ever had an anaesthetic? If so, were there any problems?
- When did she last eat and drink?
  - It is important to take a quick screening history to cover the pertinent points to be able to rapidly but safely anaesthetise a woman on labour ward. This should cover past medical history, obstetric history, drug history (including any anticoagulants or antibiotics), allergies, anaesthetic history and starvation status. This is usually followed by a brief airway assessment

b) She explains that she was diagnosed with ankylosing spondylitis two years ago. What do you want to know now? (3 marks)

- How does the disease affect her spine?
- How does it affect her mouth opening?
- Ask about any extra-articular manifestations
  - Ankylosing spondylits is a HLA-B27 mediated inflammatory disease. Patients may suffer with peripheral arthropathy, sacroilitis, inflammation of vertebral ligaments and ectopic bone formation in the spine. This can lead to nerve root compression, fractures, jaw stiffness, reduced range of movement of the spine and atlanto-axial subluxation. This has implications for the anaesthetist as it may lead to a difficult airway or technically challenging neuraxial blockade. Any pre-existing neurological deficit must be documented
  - Extra-articular complications include cardiac conduction defects, mitral valve disease, lung fibrosis, reduced chest wall compliance and uveitis

c) What do you want to know about her treatment? (3 marks)

- Does she take nonsteroidal anti-inflammatory drugs (NSAIDs)?
- Did she before getting pregnant?
- Does she take methotrexate or sulfasalazine, or were these stopped during pregnancy?
- Has she ever received anti-tumour necrosis factor (TNFα) or strong immunosuppressant treatment?
  - Ankylosing spondylitis (AS) may be treated with long term NSAIDs and this can affect renal function. Disease modifying medications such as methotrexate and sulfasalazine may cause liver impairment or blood dyscrasias and newer anti-TNFα treatments cause immunosuppression

d) She tells you that, after a previous operation, the anaesthetist told her that it was difficult for them to put a tube in her mouth and that she should always tell anaesthetists this in the future. What should you ask? (5 marks)

- What operation was she having done when this happened?
- Was it an emergency operation?
- Ask if she knows how they managed her airway e.g. did they wake her up and perform an awake fibreoptic intubation?
- Has she had any anaesthesia involving a spinal or epidural before? If so, was she told that it was difficult?

e) What do you want to ask about, given that her baby has IUGR? (2 marks)

- Does she smoke cigarettes?
- Does she drink alcohol?
  - The risk factors for IUGR may also have an impact on the anaesthetic management. Risk factors include primiparity, young or advanced age, alcohol excess, smoking and malnourishment of the mother

6. The needlephobic patient

Questions

Please take an anaesthetic history from this 54-year-old lady who is due to have a mastectomy.

a) How are you going to start the interview? (4 marks)
b) On further questioning you elicit a history of breast cancer. What details are important for you to know about the cancer diagnosis? (4 marks)
c) She tells you she has had chemotherapy. What further information is relevant? (4 marks)
d) She tells you her white cell count is low. What could you ask her about? (2 marks)
e) What other general questions are important? (2 marks)
f) You find out she has had a previous breast operation; what additional information would you like to have? (2 marks)
g) She tells you that it was fine, however she is needle phobic. What should you now ask? (2 marks)

Answers

a) How are you going to start the interview? (4 marks)
- Start by introducing yourself, confirming the patient's full name and age / date of birth. You should then explain that you are going to ask some questions to help plan the anaesthetic
- Confirm with the patient the side of the mastectomy
- Ask her why she is having the operation

b) On further questioning you elicit a history of breast cancer. What details are important for you to know about the cancer diagnosis? (4 marks)
- When was she diagnosed?
- What investigations have been performed?
- Has the cancer spread elsewhere or is it just the breast involved?
  - This is important as she may have lung or liver involvement

c) She tells you she has had chemotherapy. What further information is relevant? (4 marks)
- What chemotherapy has she had?
- How many cycles has she undergone and when was the last one?
- Does she have any long-term intravenous lines?
- Has she had any complications as a result of the chemotherapy?
  - You do not need to know exact drug regimens but the timing can influence how immunosuppressed the patient may be. If the patient has long-term IV access it may be possible to use it for induction if no other access can be found. Any indwelling lines should be aspirated before use and strict aseptic non-touch technique must be used for injection. The line should be flushed and its use documented
  - If patients have had radiotherapy, scar tissue may lead to an increase in blood loss and length of surgery. Radiotherapy near to the airway may cause scarring and distortion making intubation difficult

d) She tells you her white cell count is low. What could you ask her about? (2 marks)
- Does she feel unwell? Is she suffering from fevers, sore throat, rashes, cough, diarrhoea or any urinary symptoms?
- Has she been told that she is anaemic? Does she get out of breath on minimal exertion?
- Has she noticed that she bruises easily or has more frequent nosebleeds?
  - It is important to rule out any active infection and pancytopaenia

e) What other general questions are important? (2 marks)
- Does she have any other medical problems?
- Has she ever had an anaesthetic before? If so, for what operation(s) and were there any problems with the anaesthetic?
- What medication does she take and does she have any allergies?
- Does she smoke cigarettes or drink alcohol?

f) You find out she has had a previous breast operation; what additional information would you like to have? (2 marks)
- Did she have the operation under local or general anaesthetic?
- Were there any anaesthetic problems that she was aware of?
- Did she have any post-operative nausea and vomiting?
- Did she have an axillary node clearance at that time? If so, which side? Does she have a swollen arm as a result?
  - Axillary node clearance may lead to lymphoedema and it may be best to avoid that side for cannulation and blood pressure monitoring. She may also be anxious as a result of having

gone through a similar procedure before. The high incidence of chronic pain following mastectomy may mean that she is taking analgesics already

g) She tells you that it was fine, however she is needle phobic. What should you now ask? (2 marks)

- How was her needle phobia handled during her previous operation? Did she require a gas induction? Did they use a long line?
- What worries her in particular?
  - There is a spectrum of needle phobia from the slightly anxious, to those who would rather refuse an operation. As with all histories you need to elicit clear details. In this station your job is not to persuade the patient to have a cannula, but you do need to find out about the patient's ideas, concerns and expectations in relation to the cannula, and any measures that may be taken to make the patient more comfortable – remember the purpose of a history is to help plan your anaesthetic

This situation also comes up as a communication station. Remember, safety is paramount and it may not be appropriate to proceed with induction without intravenous access.

Options for negotiation with the patient involve putting the cannula in prior to coming to theatre in a less anxiety-provoking environment, distraction techniques and having a family member or friend present. Use of eutetic mixture of local anaesthetics (EMLA) cream or ethyl chloride spray, using the smallest gauge cannula and having the most experienced anaesthetist putting in the cannula may also help.

It would be important to explain the risks of anaesthesia without a cannula: inhalational induction is hazardous without intravenous (IV) access to give emergency drugs if required.

It would be within the patient's rights to refuse cannulation, but in an elective situation you would not be obliged to continue with the anaesthetic. In an emergency situation it would be reasonable to discuss with your consultant, and have a plan for emergency IV/intraosseous (IO) access if you did proceed with an inhalational induction, in addition to having a second anaesthetist present at induction.

7. Arterio-Venous fistula

Questions

Please take a history from this 50-year-old man who is due to have an atrioventricular (AV) fistula created on your list.
a) What are the pertinent questions to ask this patient? (4 marks)
b) What questions are you going to ask about his renal disease? (8 marks)
c) What concurrent medical problems might he have that you should ask about? (3 marks)
d) What questions do you need to ask him with respect to his airway? (5 marks)

[Handwritten notes:]

Indication for AV
→ renal failure → Cause.
    → line in situ / peritoneal dialysis
    → how long for
    → ? ↑BP
    → fluid restriction
    → ? prev renal transplant

Answers

a) What are the pertinent questions to ask this patient? (4 marks)
- What is his past medical, surgical and anaesthetic history?
- What does he know about his renal disease?

b) What questions are you going to ask about his renal disease? (8 marks)
- How long has he had kidney problems?
- Does he know what caused his kidney problems initially?
- Does he have diabetes or high blood pressure? If relevant are these currently well managed/ under control?
- How is his kidney disease managed currently? Is he on dialysis – if so how long for, what type, how often and where does it take place?
- Does he have a long-term IV line in situ? Has he had problems previously with his dialysis?
- Has he ever had a renal transplant?
- Is he fluid-restricted?
- Does he pass urine and if so how much?
  - There are many questions to ask, it is evident he has chronic renal failure; your aim is to find out how severe it is and how this will change your anaesthetic management

c) What concurrent medical problems might he have that you should ask about? (3 marks)
- Does he have a cardiovascular history? Does he have chest pain, breathing difficulties or swollen ankles?
- What is his exercise tolerance?
- Has he been told he has anaemia?

d) What questions do you need to ask him with respect to his airway? (5 marks)
- General airway questions:
  - Does he have any loose or damaged teeth?
  - Does he have any problems opening his mouth?
  - Has he had any previous anaesthetics? If so, were there any problems managing his airway?
  - When did he last have anything to eat or drink?
  - Does he suffer from acid indigestion or reflux?

Further information on patients with renal disease

Chronic renal failure is a multi-system disorder. It is diagnosed when the GFR is <35, and dialysis is indicated when the glomerular filtration rate (GFR) is <15. Care should be taken with medications that are renally excreted or nephrotoxic. In addition, fluid balance and electrolytes should be managed cautiously, and care should be taken with venous, central and arterial access. There may be impaired gastric emptying due to autonomic neuropathy and impaired immunity.

8. Fractured neck of femur

Questions

Please take a history from this 81-year-old lady who is waiting for a dynamic hip screw for a fractured neck of femur.

a) How do you start the interview? (4 marks)

b) What do you need to know about how the injury occurred? (6 marks)

c) What do you need to know about the management so far? (5 marks)

d) It seems she tripped over the rug in her sheltered housing, didn't hit her head, and pressed her buzzer for assistance. She has been given oral pain relief after she had a needle injection to numb her hip in A&E. You continue with the history. What questions do you ask about her past medical history? (2 marks)

e) You asked her if she has any problems with her heart, she says she didn't think so but one of the doctors she saw yesterday said they thought she had a murmur, she is a little anxious about this. How do you proceed? (2 marks)

f) Have you forgotten anything? (1 mark)

Answers

a) How do you start the interview? (4 marks)
- Introduce yourself
- Confirm the patient's name and date of birth
- Confirm the side of the hip fracture
- Clarify her understanding of the need for the operation

b) What do you need to know about how the injury occurred? (6 marks)
- Does she have a cardiac history that may have precipitated the fall? Did she have any symptoms prior to the fall? E.g. syncopal episodes, palpitations or chest pain
- Has she had a recent illness such as a urinary tract infection?
- Does she have a history of seizures?
- What does she remember about the fall – was it a mechanical fall?
- Did she sustain a head or neck injury?
- How long was she on the floor before she was found?
- Falls are commonly associated with head and cervical spine injuries in the elderly. She may also be at risk of rhabdomyolysis following a prolonged period on the floor

c) What do you need to know about the management so far? (5 marks)
- Is she in pain?
- How long has she been starved for? Have fluids been started?
- Does she know whether she has been started on antibiotics or any other new medications?
- Does she usually take warfarin?
- Has she had a CT scan of her head?
- You need to consider whether she has been optimised prior to the operation.

d) It seems she tripped over the rug in her sheltered housing, didn't hit her head, and pressed her buzzer for assistance. She has been given oral pain relief after she had a needle injection to numb her hip in accident and emergency (A&E). You continue with the history. What questions do you ask about her past medical history? (2 marks)
- A detailed medical, surgical and anaesthetic history should be taken
- Social and functional history
- A systems review is useful to make sure nothing has been missed

e) You asked her if she has any problems with her heart, she says she didn't think so but one of the doctors she saw yesterday said they thought she had a murmur, she is a little anxious about this. How do you proceed? (2 marks)
- Make sure you have covered her cardiac history and symptoms
- Did she have rheumatic fever as a child?
- What is her exercise tolerance?
- Has she ever had any cardiac investigations in the past?

Murmurs are relatively common in the elderly. They are significant if associated with symptoms; in this case it may have contributed to her fall. You need to consider the risk:benefit ratio of general anaesthetic versus regional anaesthetic for her operation and whether a pre-operative echocardiogram (ECHO) is warranted.

f) Have you forgotten anything? (1 mark)
- When did she last eat or drink anything
- Does she suffer from reflux?

What are pertinent questions for a dynamic hip screw (DHS)?

- Consider that the patient could have a general anaesthetic or a regional anaesthetic. Therefore, questions about medications such as warfarin, aspirin, clopidogrel and low-molecular-weight heparin (LMWH) are important. You should enquire about any lower back problems. Also you need to ask questions about previous general/regional anaesthetics and the patient's experience of them

9. Total hip replacement

Questions

You are asked to take an anaesthetic history from a 65-year-old male patient having a total hip replacement.

a) You find out the patient has osteoarthritis and this is his first operation. You are asking about his past medical history and he tells you he has some breathing problems because he used to smoke. What further questions do you need to ask? (5 marks)

b) What questions do you need to ask about his exercise tolerance/functional status? (5 marks)

c) When you take his drug history you discover he is taking amlodipine, ramipril and a low dose of bisoprolol. What questions do you need to ask? (8 marks)

d) For a patient with respiratory disease having a total hip replacement (THR), what other questions might you need to ask in order to plan your anaesthetic? (2 marks)

Answers

a) You find out the patient has osteoarthritis and this is his first operation. You are asking about his past medical history and he tells you he has some breathing problems because he used to smoke. What further questions do you need to ask? (5 marks)
- How many cigarettes per day and for how long did he smoke?
- When did he give up smoking?
- Does he have a diagnosis of chronic obstructive pulmonary disease (COPD)?
- Does he see his GP or a specialist for this?
- Is he on any medications? How often does he take them?
- Does he have problems with recurrent chest infections? Has he had any recent courses of high dose steroids?
- Has he ever been admitted to hospital for his COPD? For how long? Did he go to high dependency unit (HDU) or intensive care unit (ICU)? Did he have non-invasive (NIV) or invasive ventilation?
- Does he have any oxygen at home? Does he have home NIV?
- Is he well currently?
- Does he have a cough? Has it changed recently? Has he noticed any haemoptysis? Has he noticed any anorexia or weight loss?

b) What questions do you need to ask about his exercise tolerance/functional status? (5 marks)
- Does he ever get chest pain or shortness of breath? Does he get this at rest?
- How far is he able to walk? Does he use a stick or Zimmer frame? Is he able to leave the house?
- Is he able to climb stairs – how many?
- Is he able to cook/clean/shop/dress himself or does he require any help?
- Does he have any carers – if so how often?
  - For any chronic medical condition, particularly those that affect the respiratory or cardiovascular systems, it is important to conduct an assessment of exercise tolerance and functional status. He is likely to be limited by both his COPD and his osteoarthritis.

c) When you take his drug history you discover he is taking amlodipine, ramipril and a low dose of bisoprolol. What questions do you need to ask? (8 marks)
- In a patient with a chronic respiratory condition, especially one caused by smoking, you will already have taken a full cardiovascular history. On occasion, the drug history does uncover further issues – especially as patients don't always consider hypertension to be a medical problem
- When was he diagnosed with hypertension?
- Is this managed by his GP, or a specialist?
- How often does he see them and when was his blood pressure (BP) last checked? Is it under control?
- Does he have any ankle swelling, orthopnoea, chest pain or shortness of breath (if not already asked)
- Does he get palpitations or has he been told he has an irregular heart beat?
- Has he ever had a heart attack or stroke?
- Does he have any kidney or eye problems?
- Has he taken his medication this morning?

d) For a patient with respiratory disease having a total hip replacement (THR), what other questions might you need to ask in order to plan your anaesthetic? (2 marks)
- Does he take any blood thinning medication?
- Has he had problems with his back?
- Would he be able to lie flat if the operation was conducted under regional anaesthesia?
  - Although you are not expected to discuss general versus regional with the patient in your history station, you need to demonstrate to the examiner that you have thought of this option.

Patients with COPD

The problems in COPD mainly comprise the development of airway obstruction, mucous hyper-secretion and reduction in function of the muco-cilliary escalator. The patient is at increased risk of intra-operative laryngospasm, bronchospasm and post-operative pneumonia. It is important to opti-mise the patient either for elective or emergency theatre; this may mean a delay in surgery to recover from a cough or cold, to start antibiotics, steroids and/or inhalers, or even the use of NIV. A forced expiratory volume (FEV)1 of <1L is a poor prognostic sign in terms of respiratory secretion clearance, and increases the likelihood of requiring respiratory support post-operatively. Always consider the possibility of cor-pulmonale and consider an echocardiogram.

Further reading

Fombon, F. et al. Anaesthesia for the adult patient with rheumatoid arthritis. *BJA:CEACCP*, 6 (6): 235–9, 2006

Department of Health: Immunization against infectious disease, 2006. Available at: http://www.dh.gov.uk/prod_consum_dh/groups/dh_digitalassets/documents/digitalasset/dh_131000.pdf

Norwood, S et al. Incidence of Tracheal Stenosis and Other Late Complications After Percutaneous Tracheostomy. *Ann Surg*, 232 (2): 233–41, 2000

Regan K. et al. Tracheostomy Management. *BJA:CEACCP*, 8 (1): 31–5, 2008

Nicholson G. et al. Diabetes and the adult surgical patient. *BJA:CEACCP* Advance Access 10.1093, 2011

Gustafsson, U et al. Haemaglobin1AC as a predictor of postoperative hyperglycaemia and complications after major colorectal surgery. *Br J Surg*, 96: 1358–64, 2009

NICE SUGAR investigators. Intensive versus Conventional Glucose Control in Critically Ill Patients. *N Eng J Med*, 360: 1283–97, 2009

Joint guidelines from the Royal College of Anaesthetists and Royal College of Opthalmologists: *Local Anaesthesia for Opthalmic Surgery*, Feb 2012

Gordon H. Preoperative Assessment in ophthalmic regional anaesthesia. *BJA:CEACCP*, 6 (5): 203–6, 2006

Chung F et al. STOP questionnaire: a tool to screen patients for obstructive sleep apnoea. *Anaesthesiology*, 108: 812–21, 2008

Woodward L. et al. Ankylosing spondylitis: recent developments and anaesthetic implications. *Anaesthesia*, 64 (5): 540–8, 2009

Wen S. et al. Intrauterine growth retardation and preterm delivery: prenatal risk factors. *Gynaecology*, 162 (1): 213–18, 1990

Westbrook A, Buggy D. Anaesthesia for breast surgery *BJA:CEPD Reviews*, 3 (5): 151–4, 2003

Lewis J, Telford R. Anaesthesia for vascular surgery of the upper limb. *Contin Educ Anaesth Crit Care Pain*, (2013) doi: 10.1093/bjaceaccp/mkt044 First published online: 3 September 2013

Maxwell L, White S. Anaesthetic management of patients with hip fractures: an update. *Contin Educ Anaesth Crit Care Pain*, (2013). First published online: 26 February 2013

Bromhead, H. Total Hip Replacement: http://www.frca.co.uk/article.aspx?articleid=100977

Expand+Continuing Education in Anaesthesia, Critical Care & Painceaccp.oxfordjournals.org Grant C, Checketts M. Analgesia for primary hip and knee arthroplasty: the role of regional anaesthesia. *Contin Educ Anaesth Crit Care Pain*, 8 (2): 56–61, 2008

Chapter 4 **Communication**

Introduction

There will be one communication station in your OSCE. Although marks are rewarded for having good communication skills, being polite and using appropriate language, the majority of marks are reserved for obtaining relevant information.

This station tests knowledge of the subject and you will be expected to show your knowledge of the topic in the way you ask questions. Make sure that you test the patients understanding and check they have no further questions at the end of the station.

Typical scenarios involve explaining a procedure or complication, taking consent, or discussing treatment options.

1. Post dural puncture headache

Questions

This is Mrs Clarke. She is 24 years old and gave birth 36 hours ago. She had an epidural sited for labour. She is complaining of a headache and was seen by your consultant this morning who diagnosed a post dural puncture headache. She wants further explanation about what has happened.

a) When you introduce yourself she is visibly upset – how would you approach this and what concerns may she have? (3 marks)

b) She does not understand how an epidural can cause a headache. How would you explain a post dural puncture headache to a lay person? (3 marks)

c) She is concerned that something went wrong with the epidural. How would you handle this? (2 marks)

d) She wants to know more about treatment options. She has tried regular pain killers, keeping hydrated and drinking caffeine, as suggested by your colleague earlier that day. What information can you give her? (5 marks)

e) She says that she wants an epidural blood patch, as she cannot cope with the pain. What do you need to explain? (4 marks)

f) Performing an epidural blood patch. This is a communication station however you may still be asked to explain how the procedure is performed. (3 marks)

Answers

a) When you introduce yourself she is visibly upset – how would you approach this and what concerns may she have? (3 marks)
- Start by introducing yourself
- Show empathy for her pain and difficult situation
- Try to assess her understanding of what has happened and what exactly is upsetting her
- Is she in pain?
- Is she feeling frustrated at being unable to look after her new baby?
- Is she concerned that something has 'gone wrong' or that she has developed a serious complication?

b) She does not understand how an epidural can cause a headache. How would you explain a post dural puncture headache to a lay person? (3 marks)
- Use simple, clear language and be concise
- The brain and spinal cord are suspended in a bag filled with fluid
- During an epidural or spinal injection, the thin, outer layer of this bag can intentionally or unintentionally breeched. The hole in this bag allows the fluid to leak out
- The vast majority heal without any problems
- We think it causes a headache as certain structures in the brain are stretched and blood vessels in the brain may open up
- Over time this hole will close up, stopping the leak and the headache will resolve

c) She is concerned that something went wrong with the epidural. How would you handle this? (2 marks)
- Start by explaining that headaches are a recognised complication following an epidural
- It can help to give numbers and figures but try to present them in an easily digestible manner. About 1.5% of epidurals result in a cerebrospinal fluid leak; of those patients who have such a leak, 52% will go on to develop a headache
- It is important to tell her that post-dural-puncture headaches (PDPH)s are not usually associated with serious neurological problems
- With time the leak should gradually heal and the headache resolve

d) She wants to know more about treatment options. She has tried regular pain killers, keeping hydrated and drinking caffeine, as suggested by your colleague earlier that day. What information can you give her? (5 marks)
- It may be worth reiterating that the headache will most likely resolve spontaneously in one to 2 weeks
- You must assess how well she is able to cope at present and what support network she would have, should she go home.
- Treatment options include:
  - conservative management
  - drugs, similar to those used in the treatment of migraines (e.g. sumatriptan)
  - epidural blood patch – it is thought that epidural blood patches work by sealing off the CSF leak and causing an increase in intracranial pressure

e) She says that she wants an epidural blood patch, as she cannot cope with the pain. What do you need to explain? (4 marks)
- Here it is vital that you explain the risks, side effects and success rates for epidural blood patches
- Injection of the blood can cause backache and paraesthesia and the patient usually has to lie down for an hour after the procedure but can then return to gentle activity

- Complications are rare but include seizures, infection (meningitis/arachnoiditis), longer term nerve pain (radiculitis) and arrhythmias. Although the most senior anaesthetist available will do the procedure there is always a risk that another dural puncture can occur and the headache may get worse
- Although the blood patch is the most successful treatment available, only about 50% of patients are completely cured after one blood patch and 40% will go on to require a second blood patch

f) Performing an epidural blood patch.

This is a communication station however you may still be asked to explain how the procedure is performed. (3 marks)

- Two anaesthetists will be needed to perform the blood patch, including the most senior anaesthetist available
- A drip should be sited
- Full asepsis is established by both anaesthetists
- The epidural space is located in the usual way, usually at the space, or one space below, where the original puncture occurred
- The second anaesthetist then withdraws 40mls of blood from a peripheral vein using an aseptic technique and 10–30mls of blood is injected immediately into the epidural space. Injection should be stopped if the patient experiences radicular pain or backache
- The patient should then lie flat for an hour and refrain from heavy lifting for a few days. They should be told to seek help if they experience fevers or back pain following the procedure

2. Analgesia for an ex-intravenous drug user

Questions

This is Mr Ward, he is 40 years old. Please discuss the options for post-operative pain relief following an emergency laparotomy for acute bowel obstruction.

a) How do you start this conversation? (4 marks)

b) The patient has no allergies or significant medical problems but he immediately asks if he will be prescribed morphine. What else would you like to know? (1 mark)

c) He reveals that he is concerned, as he has previously used heroin. What else do you want to know? (8 marks)

d) He states that he does not want to be given intravenous morphine under any circumstances. How would you approach this? (3 marks)

e) He is also angry that it is written in his notes that he was an ex-drug user. How would you deal with this? (4 marks)

Answers

a) How do you start this conversation? (4 marks)
- Introduce yourself
- clearly explain that this is a forum to discuss post-operative pain relief
- establish whether the patient has any allergies
- ask about any past medical history that may influence your prescribing

b) The patient has no allergies or significant medical problems but he immediately asks if he will be prescribed morphine. What else would you like to know? (1 mark)
- Elicit his concerns about morphine. Patients may be concerned about side effects, such as nausea, sedation, constipation, or about the potential for opiate addiction

c) He reveals that he is concerned, as he has previously used heroin. What else do you want to know? (8 marks)
- When did he last use heroin?
- What treatment programs has he accessed?
- Is he taking methadone? It may be that he is taking methadone and is concerned about how this will affect the amount of analgesia he receives
- Reassure him that if he cannot take oral medication after his operation, the methadone dose will be incorporated into the amount of opiate he receives intravenously
- Reassure him that he will not be deprived of opiate medication because of his previous drug use
- A frank conversation about tolerance and dose requirements and offering him regular review by the pain team may be helpful
- He may be concerned about the potential for becoming addicted after exposure to opiates. The use of opiates in acute pain does not cause dependence or physical addiction; the euphoria felt with recreational use is not seen in the hospital setting
- The use of strong opiates will be reviewed daily and his analgesia stepped down as he recovers. Such a reduction should not elicit withdrawal symptoms, as it is likely that intravenous morphine will only be required for a short period
- This is a communication station, not a history station. It is more important to explore his concerns than ask direct questions about his drug use. However, some hard information may be useful.

d) He states that he does not want to be given intravenous morphine under any circumstances. How would you approach this? (3 marks)
- Explain that this is a major operation associated with significant levels of pain post-operatively and that poor pain relief may lead to chest infections, slower recovery and a longer hospital stay
- Opiates are the strongest analgesia available and it is unlikely that he will be unable to manage without some kind of opiate analgesia
- You could discuss regional anaesthesia and opiate sparing strategies such as co-prescription with other analgesics
- Ultimately the purpose of the discussion is to find out why he is so adamant he should not receive opiates, and to address his fears
- Explore his support network
- Offer to discuss the matter again with your consultant or a member of the pain team

e) He is also angry that it is written in his notes that he was an ex-drug user. How would you deal with this? (4 marks)

- This is testing your ability to deal with an angry patient in a calm manner – stay calm!
- Explain that medical notes are confidential and are only accessed by medical professionals directly involved in his care
- Reassure him that it is not used to label him but is an important part of his medical history as it may affect how his body reacts to medication, influence what diagnoses are more likely and highlights that certain procedures like intravenous access may be more difficult
- It may be appropriate to offer a discussion with a senior colleague about this and to make sure that the conversation is carefully documented.

3. Suxamethonium apnoea

Questions

This is Mrs Kent she is the mother of a 15-year-old boy who is currently on your intensive care unit. The patient was transferred to your care from theatre, as he required prolonged ventilation due to suxamethonium apnoea.

a) What would you initially want to find out from his mother? (3 marks)
b) She wants to know why her son needs to be on a ventilator after his operation has finished. (5 marks)
c) She is concerned that this sounds very serious – how could you reassure her? (5 marks)
d) She asks whether this will happen every time he needs an anaesthetic. What would you tell her? (3 marks)
e) She asks if she needs to tell her son's GP – what would you explain about follow up? (4 marks)

Answers

a) What would you initially want to find out from his mother? (3 marks)
- Firstly, establish what information she has been told. She will be anxious and upset. Make sure that you are sympathetic
- Reassure her that her son is being cared for
- Tell her that she will be able to visit him

b) She wants to know why her son needs to be on a ventilator after his operation has finished. (5 marks)
- Explain that you think her son has a condition called suxamethonium apnoea
- Suxamethonium is a medication used by anaesthetists to cause muscle relaxation so that patients' breathing can be taken over by a breathing machine for an operation
- Usually the effects last about 4 minutes but in a very small group of patients they are prolonged – up to several hours
- This prolonged action means that the patient's breathing must be supported until the effects of the drug have worn off
- On ICU, muscle power can be monitored and when this has normalized, he can be woken up

c) She is concerned that this sounds very serious – how could you reassure her? (5 marks)
- It is very important that this condition is recognized and all trained anaesthetists are aware of it
- There are no long term effects of this condition
- His surgery has not been affected
- He is being kept asleep whilst his muscle power returns
- He is not in any pain or discomfort

d) She asks whether this will happen every time he needs an anaesthetic. What would you tell her? (3 marks)
- Firstly, explain that there are several drugs used for muscle relaxation and that it is unlikely that this will happen with the other drugs. During routine anaesthetics suxamethonium can be avoided
- Suxamethonium is, however, the drug of choice in emergency procedures
- Her son must be aware that he has this condition, carry an alert card and inform doctors about it on future hospital admissions

e) She asks if she needs to tell her son's GP – what would you explain about follow up? (4 marks)
- Advise her that this condition does need further investigation
- The hospital will write to her GP and forward a copy of the letter to her
- It is an inherited condition, therefore she and her direct family should be tested as they may also be affected
- This will be organized at a specialized unit and this referral will be arranged by the anaesthetic team at this hospital

4. Cancellation of a paediatric case

Questions

You have been asked by your consultant to cancel a 5-year-old boy's planned tonsillectomy, as he has an upper respiratory tract infection. This is Mrs Barker, the mother of the patient.

a) How would you start the discussion? (3 marks)

b) The patient's mother says that she doesn't understand why an infection should delay surgery. How would you tackle this? (3 marks)

c) She asks if he can be rebooked for 2 days' time, as her son appears to be towards the end of his cold. How do you respond? (4 marks)

d) She is irritated that she has had to take the day off work – how do you deal with this? (6 marks)

e) She wants to talk to the surgeons – what should you say? (3 marks)

f) How would you close the discussion? (1 mark)

Answers

a) How would you start the discussion? (3 marks)
- Introduce yourself and state your role clearly
- Make sure you confirm her relationship to the patient
- Ask the mother what she has already been told
- Start by explaining that her son's operation needs to be cancelled
- Apologise for this
- Try to be empathetic – she is likely to be worried about her son undergoing surgery and the risk of delaying it

b) The patient's mother says that she doesn't understand why an infection should delay surgery. How would you tackle this? (3 marks)
- Explain that the cancellation is to make sure that her son's operation is as low-risk as possible
- When children have active respiratory tract infections they are at higher risk of breathing problems during and after anaesthesia
- Research has also shown an increased risk of bleeding following tonsillectomy in children with infections

c) She asks if he can be rebooked for 2 days' time, as her son appears to be towards the end of his cold. How do you respond? (4 marks)
- Explain that ideally 2 weeks should elapse between the end of the infection and elective surgery
- This gives the airways a chance to recover and return to normal after an infection and lowers the risk of breathing and bleeding problems
- Her son's operation will be prioritised as it has been cancelled once
- Don't make promises that you can't keep: don't offer an appointment straight after the 2 weeks are over as you are unlikely to have control over this

d) She is irritated that she has had to take the day off work – how do you deal with this? (6 marks)
- Apologise
- Reassure her that the operation will be rebooked as soon as possible
- Showing empathy for the inconvenient situation can help
- Reiterate that it is important to perform the operation when it is as safe as possible
- Give clear instructions as to how it will be rebooked
- Let her know that her son can now eat and drink

e) She wants to talk to the surgeons – what should you say? (3 marks)
- Don't be offended by this!
- Tell her that you have discussed the case with the surgical team and they agree that postponing the operation is the correct course of action
- Reassure her that a member of the surgical team will see her and her son
- Offer to have your senior colleague discuss the matter with her

f) How would you close the discussion? (1 mark)
- Finish the meeting with an apology and check that she has no further questions

5. Awake fibreoptic intubation

Questions

This is Mr Stewart. He is a 52-year-old gentleman who has previously been woken following a failed intubation for an elective laparoscopic cholecysectomy. The consultant anaesthetist has decided to proceed this time using an awake fibreoptic intubation. You are asked to explain this to the patient.

a) What are the important areas to cover? (4 marks)

b) What further information do you need from the patient? (1 mark)

c) You find out that he knows the consultant had difficulty putting the breathing tube in, they tried a few different techniques but they still couldn't see the hole for the breathing tube so they had to wake him up. He went home the same day and hasn't had any problems since. How will you explain why he needs to be intubated for this operation? (6 marks)

d) How will you explain and gain consent for a fibreoptic intubation? (6 marks)

e) How will you close the interview? (3 marks)

Answers

a) What are the important areas to cover? (4 marks)

- Explain why he needs to be intubated
- Find out what the problems were last time
- Explain what the options are this time and why we think awake fibreoptic intubation is the best option
- You need to explain what he can expect from the experience
- This station tests your ability to gain informed consent and communicate effectively using lay terminology. It is also specifically testing your knowledge about the technique of fibreoptic intubation. In general, for this type of question, you need to demonstrate an understanding of indications and contraindications for the procedure, risks and benefits to the procedure, alternative options to the proposed intervention, and varieties in technique.

b) What further information do you need from the patient? (1 mark)

- You need to try to ascertain what the patient understands from last time

c) You find out that he knows the consultant had difficulty putting the breathing tube in, they tried a few different techniques but they still couldn't see the hole for the breathing tube so they had to wake him up. He went home the same day and hasn't had any problems since. How will you explain why he needs to be intubated for this operation? (6 marks)

- Explain that unfortunately for this sort of operation there is no option for him to stay awake by using local techniques, therefore he will need a general anaesthetic
- When patients have a general anaesthetic the muscle tone in their neck relaxes, this can lead to obstruction to their breathing
- In addition, the muscles in the food pipe also relax so there is a risk of regurgitating stomach contents
- During some procedures such as laparoscopic surgery the risk of this occurring is high so we put a breathing tube in to prevent it and to protect the lungs
- Unfortunately, It seems that there were problems putting the breathing tube in last time. This can happen for a variety of reasons
- Sometimes we can predict difficulties from an airway assessment before the anaesthetic, but often we cannot predict them and problems arise once you go off to sleep. We are keen to avoid problems this time, and that is what I am going to talk to you about today

d) How will you explain and gain consent for a fibreoptic intubation? (6 marks)

- Explain that it is very rare not to be able to visualise the vocal cords, but because it happened previously there is a high chance of it happening again. If we failed to insert the tube correctly this could lead to a lack of oxygen being delivered to you and that can have very serious consequences
- We think therefore that a different technique is needed. This is called awake fibreoptic intubation
- We will use local anaesthetic applied to your nose and to the back of your throat to numb these areas
- While you are awake we will pass a thin tube with a small camera at the end through your nose to visualise the hole between the vocal cords that we need to pass the breathing tube through
- We will then pass the small tube through your nose into the back of your throat, over the tube with the camera at the end. We can see what is happening throughout
- You will be sitting up whilst this is happening, and attached to the same monitoring as if you were having a general anaesthetic

- We can use medication to make you more relaxed, and these often make you less likely to remember the procedure afterwards
- However, we will not let you go to sleep because should this occur there is a risk that the airway would collapse and we wouldn't be able to get enough oxygen into your lungs
- This process of awake fibreoptic intubation can be uncomfortable but it shouldn't be painful. If it is then you will be able to let us know and we can apply more local anaesthetic to make you more comfortable
- We feel this is the safest option for in your case
- As soon as the tube has been passed safely into your airway we will send you off to sleep using drugs injected into a drip in your arm
- When we wake you up at the end of the operation we have to make sure that you are fully awake before we take the tube out – again this may be something you are aware of or remember, it shouldn't last for very long, and again it is for your safety
- It is a commonplace procedure and is very safe. The risks include being unable to insert the tube (although this is very rare), discomfort, bleeding, damage to your nose, mouth, throat and trachea

e) How will you close the interview? (3 marks)

- It is always important to check the patient has understood what you have told them
- Find out if he has any questions
- Check that he is happy with the anaesthetic plan

Further information

The main indications for an awake intubation are an anticipated or known difficult airway situation (difficult intubation and/or difficult facemask ventilation). It may also have a role in emergency situations to reduce the risk of aspiration, to prevent cardiovascular collapse, and to minimise mobilisation of the C-spine. Absolute and relative contra-indications include patient refusal, coagulopathy, an already partially obstructed airway and allergy to local anaesthetics. Options for anaesthetising the airway during awake fibreoptic intubation include topical cocaine, prilocaine or lidocaine (with or without a vasoconstrictor such as phenylephrine) or lidocaine used for nerve blocks.

The nose, pharynx and larynx need to be anaesthetised; pastes, sprays, nebulisers, trans-tracheal puncture and superior laryngeal nerve blocks can all be used effectively depending on user preference. Most anaesthetists use an IV antisaliogogue such as glycopyrrolate, and a nasal vasoconstrictor (e.g. xylometazoline) for optimum viewing conditions.

Sedation can also be used with extreme caution by experienced technicians (to ensure verbal contact throughout), for example a midazolam bolus or TCI propofol or remifentanil. Complications include failure, bleeding, haematoma, laryngospasm and local anesthetic toxicity.

6. Awareness

Questions

This is Miss Turner. She is a 35-year-old lady having a laparoscopic cholecystectomy. She is worried because she was aware during an emergency caesarean section 3 years ago.

a) What further information would you like to have? (7 marks)
b) What will you explain to her about awareness? (8 marks)
c) What else will you offer? (3 marks)
d) How will you close the conversation? (2 marks)

Answers

a) What further information would you like to have? (7 marks)
- You firstly need to know more about her experience of awareness - what exactly does she remember?
- You need to ask specifically about awareness at induction, intra-operative awareness, or awareness during emergence?
- Did she feel pain during the operation?
- You want to find out whether she had any follow up care – did she speak to anyone i.e. an anesthetist about it afterwards, has she had any counselling since?
- Is she still suffering, for example with nightmares?
- You also need to find out exactly what her concerns are for this anaesthetic – that it will happen again, she may be too scared to have an anaesthetic, she may be scared of feeling pain?
- Make sure you are empathetic

b) What will you explain to her about awareness? (8 marks)
- Firstly, it will be important to apologise to her for the experience she had last time, and to demonstrate empathy in understanding how traumatic the experience must have been
- You can go on to explain that awareness under anaesthetic is rare.
- Explain that it is more likely in emergency situations, in obstetric anaesthesia and with difficult airways
- You can explain that it would be very unlikely for this experience to be repeated in a controlled environment for an elective procedure in an otherwise well person such as herself
- It is worth explaining that we take precautionary measures in **all** patients to limit the risk of awareness including giving a calculated dose of anaesthetic agent, monitoring the amount of anaesthetic the patient is receiving, and monitoring vital signs that would indicate pain or awareness
- Explain that there is always an anaesthetist present
- Explain that she will be monitored throughout the operation
- You may want to mention the use of bispectral index monitoring

c) What else will you offer? (3 marks)
- You should explain that you will inform the consultant who will be responsible for her anaesthetic care. You should always offer the chance to speak to a consultant prior to her general anaesthetic
- Explain that everything has been documented, and you can send a letter to her GP about the previous events
- You can offer counselling prior to this general anaesthetic, and to help her deal with residual trauma from the previous anaesthetic

d) How will you close the conversation? (2 marks)
- Check understanding
- Ask if she has any further questions

Further information

Awareness can be *explicit* (conscious awareness with recall of actual events, with or without pain) or *implicit* (an apparent perception during anaesthesia with post-operative sequelae, such as poor sleep, without conscious awareness or recall). Explicit awareness may be confused with awareness during emergence, or delirium/dreaming during the recovery phase – details of recall should be clarified and, in some circumstances, it may be appropriate to reassure patients if this is evidently the case. The risk of awareness is higher in emergencies (especially obstetrics and trauma), difficult airways and use of total intravenous anaesthesia (TIVA). It can also be due to technical issues or human error.

7. Child refusing surgery

Questions

You are asked to speak to the Mrs. Wilson. She is the mother of a 14-year-old boy who has just refused to walk into the anaesthetic room prior to having a dental extraction. He was the first patient on the morning list. He had gone back to sit with his mother, and is now with one of the nurses.

a) What are the major issues that may arise during this interview? (4 marks)

b) How will you start the conversation? (5 marks)

c) She explains she didn't realise he was quite so anxious, but it is really important he has the operation done today as she has taken time off work. How will you manage her concerns and expectations? (3 marks)

d) She is obviously frustrated and says that both she and he have signed the consent form so 'can't we just put him to sleep'. How will you deal with the ethical and legal implications? (5 marks)

e) How will you negotiate a solution? (3 marks)

Answers

a) What are the major issues that may arise during this interview? (4 marks)

- The primary concern is obviously for the child, who may be very anxious and upset. The same is true of the mother
- You may need to de-escalate (or at least prevent escalation) of an emotionally charged situation
- You also need to try to formulate a plan with the child and the mother in order to facilitate the operation. This will require eliciting the patient's and mother's concerns and finding a practical solution within the limits and restrictions of what is realistically achievable in the context of an operating list
- In addition, you are being tested on your knowledge of ethical and legal guidelines regarding consent in paediatric patients

b) How will you start the conversation? (5 marks)

- Introduce yourself
- Confirm the identity of the person you are speaking with, and their relationship to the patient
- Start by 'setting the scene' or introducing the conversation you are about to have; this may involve reiterating some of the information given to you on the instruction sheet
- The next important step is to find out the other person's perception of the situation
- Show that you understand that the situation is difficult and that you want to help

c) She explains she didn't realise he was quite so anxious, but it is really important he has the operation done today as she has taken time off work. How will you manage her concerns and expectations? (3 marks)

- Empathise with his anxiety and her frustration
- Show understanding – anxiety is a common reaction to having an anaesthetic/operation – children have the same fears of needles, going to sleep, pain, and waking up that adults do
- Offer to talk to her son about the anaesthetic and the surgery
- Discuss the possibility of medication to make him more relaxed
- Offer a slot later in the morning if possible
- Explain that if he continues to refuse then surgery may have to be postponed
- It is always important to apologise and empathise, this will help to build rapport and de-escalate the situation. Aim to offer a realistic and practical solution to the problem; but do not offer something you cannot deliver; you may not be able to proceed with the operation today.

d) She is obviously frustrated and says that both she and he have signed the consent form so 'can't we just put him to sleep'. How will you deal with the ethical and legal implications? (5 marks)

- Again empathise with the mother
- Explain that with any un-cooperative child, particularly in an elective situation, it is not really in the child's best interests to proceed completely against their will
- It can cause future emotional and behavioural problems, and long-term fears of hospitals/anaesthesia/surgery
- It is especially difficult in a young adult who would have to be forcibly restrained to be anaesthetised – this would be very traumatic and is certainly not the safest way of conducting an anaesthetic
- Explain that legally, if he is judged to have full capacity, he can consent for his operation, sign a consent form, and he can withdraw his consent at any time. As a child, he cannot refuse treatment that is in his best interest, but it would be unethical to restrain him in this elective situation as there are other options available such as postponing the operation

e) How will you negotiate a solution? (3 marks)
- Offer to discuss the anaesthetic with him, with her present
- Offer methods of making it less stressful e.g. EMLA cream to numb his hand before cannulation, or a 'premed'
- Explain that mum can come to the anaesthetic room if she thinks that will help
- Discuss the option of having one of the nurses spend some time with him and being present in the anaesthetic room, and offer a distraction such as a book to read
- Offer to rearrange the operation with a plan to give sedative medication next time around
- Always offer mum the opportunity to talk to a consultant if she wishes and make sure you have answered all of her questions before you close the interview
- You could mention play therapists or referral to a psychologist if having the operation still remains unacceptable to the child

Further information

Uncooperative children are commonly encountered in anaesthetic practice. The importance of the pre-operative visit cannot be underestimated in allaying the fears of both the child and parents. It is important to explain, in a non-threatening manner, to both the child, and the family member, what they can expect. Sedation can be considered in children who are obviously going to be uncooperative. It is important to explain to parents that gentle restraint is occasionally required to facilitate siting a cannula, or during an inhalational induction. It can help to explain to mum or dad how they can help by tightly hugging their child with the child's arm behind their back during cannula insertion. This is best done before they come into the anaesthetic room.

In many situations it is advisable for a parent to accompany their child to the anaesthetic room – although there are occasions when this could make the experience more fraught if the parents are very anxious. A friendly nurse and distraction techniques can help. If children are very uncooperative or even combative, then forceful restraint can cause them long-term emotional and behavioural problems. This is not justified in the elective situation, and every effort should be made to avoid a stressful situation.

In England, children over the age of 16 (or younger if they are deemed competent) can legally consent to treatment but they must be over 18 to refuse treatment which is felt to be in their best interests. In Scotland a competent child over the age of 16 may refuse treatment.

8. Needle phobia

Questions

This is Miss Mortimer; she is a 28–year-old woman who you have been asked to assess prior to her tibial nailing. She is terrified of needles and has refused to have blood taken. She is otherwise fit and well.

a) What are the major issues that may arise during this interview? (2 marks)

b) How are you going to start this conversation? (3 marks)

c) You discover that she finds needles painful, she doesn't like the thought of having a cannula left in her vein, and she really doesn't want one. How will you negotiate these issues? (6 marks)

d) She asks if there is any way that she can go to sleep without the cannula. How will you respond? (6 marks)

e) Can you take the cannula out before I wake up? (1 mark)

f) She absolutely refuses to have pre-operative blood tests or a cannula before she is anaesthetised. How would you manage this situation? (2 marks)

Answers

a) What are the major issues that may arise during this interview? (2 marks)

- The problematic areas for communication that may arise in this scenario include managing an anxious patient, which often involves needing to give reassurance without making false promises, and negotiation
- In terms of testing your knowledge and experience this station is concerned with your ability to consider management options for needle phobic patients whilst providing a safe anaesthetic within the limits of your competence

b) How are you going to start this conversation? (3 marks)

- You should start by introducing yourself to the patient
- Confirm that you are here to talk about her fear of needles
- Try to ascertain exactly what she is frightened of

c) You discover that she finds needles painful, she doesn't like the thought of having a cannula left in her vein, and she really doesn't want one. How will you negotiate these issues? (6 marks)

- Empathise with her about her fears to build rapport
- Explain the techniques commonly employed for needle phobic patients such as EMLA cream, using a very small cannula or needle, and having the most senior anaesthetist insert the cannula
- Explain that it is not always necessary to have pre-operative blood tests, but in her case we would be checking for anaemia, and checking her blood group in case she requires a transfusion. Explain that it is safest to do this
- Offer for her to have a friend or relative come with her into the anaesthetic room
- You may offer a sedative medication pre-operatively
- Explain that the cannula itself is not a needle and once the cannula is in, anaesthetic can be given immediately

d) She asks if there is any way that she can go to sleep without the cannula. How will you respond? (6 marks)

- Explain inhalational induction
- Explain that inhalational inductions come with risks, even more so in adults as it takes longer to go to sleep and they are more prone to having irritated airways. This airway irritation means that the airways close up and it becomes difficult to get oxygen into the lungs
- In this emergency situation intravenous medication is required to resolve the problem quickly, and it takes time to put in a cannula.
- Therefore, this technique is not advised in adults
- This may be considered only in people into whom it would be easy to insert cannula in the event of an emergency
- Explain that this needs to be done by a senior anaesthetist
- This is a semi-elective operation and patient safety is paramount. It is important to convey the various options for induction of anaesthesia for full informed consent, but it is also our responsibility to explain the risks to explain the considerations for patient safety that we have to make.

e) Can you take the cannula out before I wake up? (1 mark)

- Again this is not advisable due to the risks of airway problems arising during emergence and in recovery

f) She absolutely refuses to have pre-operative blood tests or a cannula before she is anaesthetised. How would you manage this situation? (2 marks)

- Explain that it is completely within her rights to refuse a cannula and bloods, but that it would be a consultant anaesthetist's decision as to whether they would be happy to proceed with the procedure without a cannula
- Explain that you will ask a consultant to speak with her.

9. Jehovah's Witness and refusal of blood products

Questions

This is Mrs. Jones. She is a Jehovah's Witness and is due to have a total hip replacement. Her pre-operative haemoglobin is 72g/L.

a) What questions do you need to ask this patient about her acceptance of blood products? (6 marks)
b) How will you explain the risks of refusing blood products to this patient? (6 marks)
c) How will you explain options for pre-optimisating the patient prior to surgery? (4 marks)
d) What other information would you want to know about this patient's medical history in order to plan your anaesthetic? (3 marks)
e) What post-operative plan will you make with the patient? (1 mark)

Answers

a) What questions do you need to ask this patient about her acceptance of blood products? (6 marks)
- Do not make any assumptions as to the patient's understanding of blood products or her acceptance/refusal of them
- Ask specifically whether she would accept fractions of blood and clotting factors such as packed red cells, fresh frozen plasma and platelet.
- Check whether the patient would accept recombinant factor VII, and be prepared to explain what this is
- Ask if she would accept intra-operative cell salvage
- Clarify whether, in a life or death situation, the patient would rather die than accept blood products
- Does she have an advance directive? If not, advise her to make one and explain that she will need to sign documents outlining exactly what she will accept

b) How will you explain the risks of refusing blood products to this patient? (6 marks)
- Obviously you need to display respect for the patient's beliefs but you must also ensure she is fully informed about the risks prior to surgery
- An explanation about the role of blood in carrying oxygen around the body and allowing our organs to work effectively is advisable. You can further explain that surgery puts extra strain on our bodies and therefore all organs have a higher oxygen demand than normal
- Further explanation that low blood levels can cause heart failure, heart attacks, strokes and, in extreme circumstances, cardiac arrest is important as this conveys the serious risks involved
- While being polite and avoiding being dramatic, make sure the patient is aware that refusing blood or blood products may result in her death
- Specific to this scenario is the importance of explaining that hip surgery carries a high risk of blood loss both in theatre and after surgery
- You can explain how having a low haemoglobin level can make people feel tired, dizzy, and short of breath although it is possible to manage these symptoms conservatively

c) How will you explain options for pre-optimisating the patient prior to surgery? (4 marks)
- It is important that you explain the need to treat her anaemia prior to the operation. This may include investigations to find the cause of the anaemia.
- Explain the use of oral iron and the option of IV iron if oral iron is ineffective
- Erythropoietin could also be considered

d) What other information would you want to know about this patient's medical history in order to plan your anaesthetic? (3 marks)
- Your task is not to take a history, but you may want to quickly find out some more information such as why the patient is anaemic, if she is on any treatment for anaemia, whether she takes any anticoagulants or antiplatelet agents
- You may be thinking ahead to your anaesthetic plan, and consider risk factors for hypotensive anaesthesia, acute hypervolaemic haemodilution or regional anaesthesia as strategies for reducing blood loss. Ask if the patient is hypertensive or has any cardiovascular history, or any back problems

e) What post-operative plan will you make with the patient? (1 mark)
- You may discuss post-operative management on a high dependency or intensive care unit

Further reading

Sudheer P, Stacey M. Anaesthesia for awake intubation. *BJA CEPD Reviews*, 3 (4): 120–3, 2003

Hardman J, Aitkinhead A. Awareness during anaesthesia. *Contin Educ Anaesth Crit Care Pain*, 5 (6): 183–6. 2005

Tan L, Meakin P Continuing Education in Anaesthesia, Critical Care & Painceaccp.oxfordjournals.org. Anaesthesia for the uncooperative child. *Contin Educ Anaesth Crit Care Pain*, 10 (2): 48–52, 2001

Chapter 5 **Examination**

Introduction

In the OSCE there is one examination station. Typically, you will be required to examine one system and then asked questions afterwards. There will be actors, not patients in the OSCE so they should not have any positive findings!

Start the station by introducing yourself, explaining what you are going to do and asking permission to examine the actor. Make sure that they are positioned and exposed appropriately.

Do not be put off if the examiners only ask you to perform 'a bit of' your examination. For example, you may be asked just to examine the precordium rather than performing a full cardiovascular examination. This is because time is limited and you must be slick in order to have time to answer questions afterwards that will score you marks. Be ready to explain how you would 'complete an examination' if you had more time.

Be aware that sometimes you may be asked to perform an examination on a mannequin, for example in a trauma scenario.

Practice performing your examinations on friends so that you are slick, and can get through the important points in a few minutes.

1. Cranial nerve examination

Questions

This is Mrs. Talbot – she had an epidural sited 24 hours ago for labour and has since delivered. For the past 2 hours she has been complaining of a headache and blurred vision. Please examine cranial nerves II to XII. You need not perform fundoscopy.

a) How would you start the station? (1 mark)
b) What 4 tests would you perform to assess CN II (the optic nerve)? (2 marks)
c) How is the pupillary light reflex is controlled? (2 marks)
d) What are the signs of Horner's syndrome? (2 marks)
e) Examine the movements of the eyes. (1 mark)
f) How would a IV nerve palsy present? (1 mark)
g) How are the rest of the eye movements controlled? (2 marks)
h) Test the function of the trigeminal nerve. (2 marks)
i) Test the facial nerve. (2 marks)
j) Test nerves IX to XII. (3 marks)
k) Test her hearing. (2 marks)

Answers

a) How would you start the station? (1 mark)
- Introduce yourself and explain that you would like to examine the nerves supplying her head and face

b) What 4 tests would you perform to assess CN II (the optic nerve)? (2 marks)
- Visual acuity – ask if she has noticed a change in her vision. See if she can read what is written on a piece of paper (or use a Snellen chart if available), testing each eye and making sure she is using any glasses that she normally wears
- Visual fields – sitting opposite the patient, get her to cover one eye and move your finger into the superior and inferior quadrants of the temporal and nasal fields. Repeat for the other eye
- Pupillary response – test both the direct and consensual response. Also perform the swinging light test, shining a light between the two pupils to look for a relative afferent pupillary defect
- Accommodation reflex – get the patient to look into the distance then at your finger held close to their face. Constriction of the pupils should occur

c) How is the pupillary light reflex is controlled? (2 marks)
- The afferent nerve is the optic nerve (II)
- This integrates at the Edinger-Westphal nucleus and produces a bilateral response through the parasympathetic nerve fibres of the oculomotor nerve (III)
- This stimulates the ciliary ganglion to cause constriction of the pupillary sphincter

d) What are the signs of Horner's syndrome? (2 marks)

All symptoms are ipsilateral.
- Partial ptosis (levetor palpebrae is innervated by both the oculomotor nerve and sympathetic fibres)
- Miosis (sympathetic innervation to the ciliary ganglion causes pupillary dilation therefore interruption of this causes unopposed constriction)
- Anhydrosis
- Enopthalmos (due to lack of innervation to the tarsus muscles)

e) Examine the movements of the eyes. (1 mark)
- Test the movements in all 4 directions, including superior and inferior gaze whilst looking laterally (i.e. in an 'H' pattern)

f) How would a IV nerve palsy present? (1 mark)
- The trochlear nerve supplies the superior oblique muscle, which depresses the eye when it is fully adducted – this movement would not be possible

g) How are the rest of the eye movements controlled? (2 marks)
- The oculomotor nerve supplies all the other muscles except the lateral rectus, which is supplied by the abducens nerve (VI)

h) Test the function of the trigeminal nerve. (2 marks)
- Sensory – test sensation to light touch in the ophthalmic, maxillary, mandibular distributions. Offer to demonstrate the corneal reflex (afferent V1 and efferent facial via orbicularis oculi)
- Motor – test the muscles of mastication by asking the patient to clench their teeth

i) Test the facial nerve. (2 marks)
- Motor – test the muscles of facial expression
- Sensory – ask about changes in taste – the chorda tympani supplies taste to the anterior two thirds of the tongue

j) Test nerves IX to XII. (3 marks)
- The glossopharyngeal and vagus nerves are usually examined together – offer to demonstrate the gag reflex (afferent sensation of the pharynx is supplied by IX, and efferent movement

of the pharynx by X). You could ask if any she has noticed any change in her speech or swallowing

- The accessory nerve innervates the sternocleidomastoid and trapezius. Test this by getting her to shrug her shoulders and turn her head against resistance
- The hypoglossal nerve supplies motor function to the tongue. Any deviation on protrusion would indicate a lesion on the side the deviation is towards

k) Test her hearing. (2 marks)

- Ask about any change in her hearing
- Rinne's test – hold a vibrating tuning fork next to the auditory meatus (conduction in air) then place it on the mastoid process (conduction through bone). It is positive if it is loudest in air and this is normal. If bone conduction is louder, it is suggestive of conductive hearing loss. In sensorineural loss, both bone and air conduction are decreased so the test may still be positive
- Weber's test – a tuning fork is placed on the middle of the patient's forehead. Diminished perception in one ear indicates sensorineural loss in that ear. Increased perception in one ear indicates a conductive loss in the affected ear

2. Lower limb neurological examination

Questions

Mrs. Lloyd had a spinal anaesthetic for a gynaecological operation yesterday and is now complaining of a numb patch on her right leg. Please perform a neurological examination of her lower limbs.

a) How would you start the examination? (1 mark)
b) What features would you look for on inspection? (2 marks)
c) You ask her to stand – what do you want her to do? (2 marks)
d) How would you examine tone and what abnormalities of tone would you expect if there was a compressive vertebral canal haematoma? (2 marks)
e) Test her power and give it a score. (2 marks)
f) What nerve roots are required for normal hip extension and flexion? (2 marks)
g) How would you test co-ordination? (2 marks)
h) Test her reflexes – which nerve roots are involved? (2 marks)
i) Test sensation to light touch. What would you expect to find if she had a lesion affecting L5? (2 marks)
j) Which other modalities should you test? (2 marks)
k) How would you complete the examination? (1 mark)

Answers

a) How would you start the examination? (1 mark)
- Introduce yourself; explain what you are about to do. Ask permission to expose the patient's legs and check that she is positioned correctly

b) What features would you look for on inspection? (2 marks)
- Look for any pressure areas that could have resulted from being in the lithotomy position
- Look for any wasting or fasciculation that could indicate a chronic neurological problem
- See if her legs are positioned normally
- Are there are any scars

c) You ask her to stand – what do you want her to do? (2 marks)
- Romberg's test – ask her to stand with her feet together and to close her eyes. Support her whilst you do this and look for any unsteadiness A positive test indicates a problem with proprioception, or cerebellar pathology
- Gait – ask if she can walk across the cubicle and look for any abnormalities of gait

d) How would you examine tone and what abnormalities of tone would you expect if there was a compressive vertebral canal haematoma? (2 marks)
- Testing tone – passive movement will give an indication of tone
- Testing for clonus – rapid dorsiflexion at the ankle will elicit clonus Greater than 4 beats is considered abnormal and is an indication of an upper motor neurone lesion
- A vertebral canal haematoma would cause a lower motor neurone lesion therefore you would expect the patient's legs to be hypotonic

e) Test her power and give it a score. (2 marks)
- Test power using a systematic method of flexion and extension at the major joints of the lower limbs including the great toe
- Compare left with right for each movement
  - The most common scoring system is the MRC (Medical Research Council) scale:
    - 0 – no muscle contraction
    - 1 – contraction is visible but not enough power to move the joint
    - 2 – movement can occur at the joint when gravity is eliminated
    - 3 – movement can overcome gravity but not resistance from the examiner
    - 4 – movement can overcome some resistance from the examiner
    - 5 – full and normal power against resistance

f) What nerve roots are required for normal hip extension and flexion? (2 marks)
- extension – L4/5
- flexion – L2/3

g) How would you test co-ordination? (2 marks)
- Careful explanation is required for this to be done quickly and effectively. Ask the patient to touch their left knee with their right toe, slide the toe down to their ankle then lift their leg to touch your outstretched finger. Repeat three times and with the other leg
- Ask the patient to tap the soles of their feet in time against your hands

h) Test her reflexes – which nerve roots are involved? (2 marks)
- Explain to the patient what you are doing
- Knee jerk – tap the patella tendon of the relaxed limb. This tests L3/4.
- Ankle jerk – flex the knee, dorsiflex the ankle and slightly laterally rotate the leg then tap the Achilles tendon. This tests S1
- Plantar (Babinski) reflex – an upgoing plantar would suggest an upper motor neurone lesion

i) Test sensation to light touch. What would you expect to find if she had a lesion affecting L5? (2 marks)
  - If there is cotton wool available use this, if not use your finger. Try to test all the dermatomes from L2 to S1 and test each dermatome bilaterally
  - A lesion affecting L5 would lead to hypoaesthesia of the skin over the dorsum of the foot (excluding the lateral foot), lateral lower leg and great toe

j) Which other modalities should you test? (2 marks)
  - Proprioception and vibration – testing dorsal column function
  - Pinprick and temperature – testing spinothalamic function

k) How would you complete the examination? (1 mark)
  - You could ask to examine the site of the spinal injection to look for any swelling or erythema
  - You could ask about perineal sensation and bladder and bowel symptoms to help exclude cauda equina syndrome

3. ATLS primary survey

Questions

You are in the emergency department and are asked to perform a primary survey on this patient who was in a road traffic accident.

a) What do you assess first? (2 marks)

b) The patient is able to speak and there is no obvious trauma to the face. How do you stabilise the cervical spine? (2 marks)

c) You move on to assessing the patient's breathing. What are the important steps in doing this? (5 marks)

d) Name 4 life threatening traumatic injuries to the chest. (2 marks)

e) What signs would make you suspect a tension pneumothorax? (4 marks)

f) How would you assess the patient's circulation? (3 marks)

g) What else should you do during the primary survey? (2 marks)

Answers

a) What do you assess first? (2 marks)
- The airway must be assessed – ask the patient their name and see if they are able to vocalise. Listen for any snoring or abnormal sounds
- This should be done at the same time as ensuring in-line cervical spine stabilisation

b) The patient is able to speak and there is no obvious trauma to the face. How do you stabilise the cervical spine? (2 marks)

All of the following are required to ensure adequate spinal immobilisation:
- Semi-rigid collar
- Head blocks or sandbags
- Spinal board
- Taping of the forehead and collar to the spinal board in the neutral position

c) You move on to assessing the patient's breathing. What are the important steps in doing this? (5 marks)
- Ensure the patient is receiving high flow oxygen via a facemask with reservoir bag (this is a spontaneously ventilating patient)
- Examine the chest for equal expansion, any obvious injuries or paradoxical movements. Also look for any obvious cyanosis and count the respiratory rate
- Palpation – ensure equal chest expansion, feel for any crepitus that may indicate subcutaneous emphysema or rib fractures. Palpate the trachea and comment on any deviation
- Percussion – percuss each side of the chest at the apex, mid zone and base
- Auscultate – listen to each side of the chest at the apex, mid zone, base and in the axillary area

d) Name 4 life threatening traumatic injuries to the chest. (2 marks)

Any four of:
- tension pneumothorax
- open pneumothorax
- massive haemothorax
- flail chest with pulmonary contusions
- cardiac tamponade

e) What signs would make you suspect a tension pneumothorax? (4 marks)

Any 4 of:
- Increased respiratory rate
- Cyanosis
- Decrease chest expansion on the affected side
- Tracheal deviation away from the affected side
- Hyper-resonance on percussion of the affected side
- Absence of breath sounds on the affected side
- Distension of neck veins
- Circulatory collapse

f) How would you assess the patient's circulation? (3 marks)
- Look for any obvious sources of external bleeding and act to control any haemorrhage.
- Inspect the patient's colour
- Assess the pulse – rate, rhythm and character
- Find out the blood pressure
- Check capillary refill time

g) What else should you do during the primary survey? (2 marks)
- Disability – Determine the patient's level of consciousness using the Glasgow coma scale (GCS) and look for a pupillary response
- Exposure – fully examine the patient but keep them warm

4. Airway examination

Questions

Mr Jones is due to have elective surgery today. Please examine his airway.

a) How do you start the examination? (1 mark)
b) What features on inspection would make you anticipate a problematic airway? (4 marks)
c) What manoeuvres would you ask the patient to perform and what are you looking for? (6 marks)
d) You notice a mass in the anterior triangle of his neck. Describe how you would examine his neck. (4 marks)
e) If this was a thyroid mass what other systems would you want to examine? (3 marks)
f) What investigations would you request for this patient? (2 marks)

Answers

a) How do you start the examination? (1 mark)
   - Introduce yourself and explain what you are going to do
b) What features on inspection would make you anticipate a problematic airway? (4 marks)
   - Obesity
   - Short neck
   - Receding jaw
   - Abnormal dentition
   - Facial hair
   - Dysmorphic features or other evidence of congenital syndromes such as Pierre-Robin syndrome
   - Evidence of other systemic disease that may affect the airway e.g. rheumatoid deformities or exopthalmos
   - Neck masses or scars

The Wilson's score is out of 10. A score of 0–2 is allocated to each of 5 criteria (patient weight, head and neck movement, buck teeth, receding mandible and jaw movement). A score of 4 or more predicts 90% of difficult intubations.

c) What manoeuvres would you ask the patient to perform and what are you looking for? (6 marks)
   - Open your mouth (and then protrude your tongue)
     - Inter-incisor distance of <3cm predicts a difficult airway
     - Mallampati score
     - Assess dentition
     - Identify macroglossia
   - Bring your lower jaw in front of your top teeth
     - Inability to protrude the jaw is thought to be a risk factor for difficult intubation
   - Extend your neck
     - A thyromental distance of <6cm when the neck is extended is predictive of a difficult intubation
     - A sternomental distance of <12cm is also thought to be predictive
d) You notice a mass in the anterior triangle of his neck. Describe how you would examine his neck. (4 marks)
   - Look at the neck and describe the position and size of the mass and its relations to other structures
   - Ask the patient to protrude their tongue and look for any movement of the mass (movement would suggest a thyroglossal cyst)
   - Ask the patient to raise their arms and look for venous engorgement which may suggest SVC obstruction (Pemberton's sign)
   - Ask about any vocal changes
   - Stand behind the patient and palpate the mass – ask them to swallow whilst palpating the mass
   - Palpate for any lymphadenopathy in the neck
   - Percuss the sternum to elicit any retrosternal extension
   - Listen for a thyroid bruit
e) If this was a thyroid mass what other systems would you want to examine? (3 marks)
   - Cardiovascular – hyperthyroid patients may be tachycardic and have an arrhythmia. They are also at risk of high output cardiac failure

- Neurological – the patient may have a tremor and be hyperreflexic.
- Eyes – exophthalmos, lid lag and ophthalmoplegia can occur

The patient may be hyper-, hypo- or euthyroid. The signs of hyperthyroidism are generally the easiest to elicit.

f) What investigations would you request for this patient? (2 marks)

- A CT scan of the neck and thorax would help to diagnose the likely origin of the mass, to assess airway calibre and position, and to look for retrosternal extension
- A nasoendoscopy would be helpful to ensure the recurrent laryngeal nerve was not currently affected and causing vocal cord pathology. It will also indicate how easy the glottis will be to visualise at laryngoscopy
- Thyroid function tests would determine whether the patient needed medical management prior to surgery
- An ECG to assess for arrhythmias and LVH

5. Cardiovascular examination (1): murmurs

Questions

This is Mrs Cooper. She fractured her right hip yesterday following a 'mechanical fall'. The junior doctor clerking noted a systolic murmur and has requested an ECHO but it hasn't been performed yet. Please examine her cardiovascular system.

a) What comments might you make on the patient's general appearance? (5 marks)
b) Before you examine the precordium what clinical signs could help to distinguish between systolic murmurs? (4 marks)
c) How would you distinguish between the systolic murmurs of aortic stenosis and mitral regurgitation? (6 marks)
d) What further investigations would you request? (3 marks)
e) She is diagnosed as having mitral regurgitation – what would your perioperative haemodynamic goals be? (2 marks)

Answers

a) What comments might you make on the patient's general appearance? (5 marks)
- Does she look well or unwell?
- Is she comfortable at rest or are they in pain or short of breath?
- Pallor or cyanosis
- Clubbing or nicotine-stained hands
- Osler's nodes or Janeway lesions (suggestive of infective endocarditis)

b) Before you examine the precordium what clinical signs could help to distinguish between systolic murmurs? (4 marks)
- Assessment of the pulse: You may find the patient is in atrial fibrillation, which is very common in mitral valve disease. A slow-rising pulse is characteristic of severe aortic stenosis
- Assessment of the blood pressure: you may find a narrow pulse pressure with aortic stenosis

c) How would you distinguish between the systolic murmurs of aortic stenosis and mitral regurgitation? (6 marks)
- The murmur of aortic stenosis is usually audible all over the precordium, including the apex. It is usually loud, harsh and high pitched. It is an 'ejection' systolic murmur. It radiates to the carotids and may cause a thrill
- The murmur of mitral regurgitation is pan-systolic. It is usually loud and blowing. It is best heard at the apex, and radiates towards the axilla. The apex beat can be forceful and displaced. You may hear a third heart sound

d) What further investigations would you request? (3 marks)
- 12-lead ECG
- Echocardiogram (ECHO)
- Chest X-ray

As with all cardiac murmurs their significance peri-operatively is largely dependent on the degree of compromise to the patient, so a thorough cardiovascular history and functional assessment is required. In addition to this, all patients require an ECG and chest X-ray. Any abnormalities in the history or on the ECG would prompt an echocardiogram. In the case of mitral regurgitation, asymptomatic patients usually tolerate non-cardiac surgery well.

e) She is diagnosed as having mitral regurgitation – what would your perioperative haemodynamic goals be? (2 marks)
- High-normal heart rate
- Adequate pre-load
- Low systemic vascular resistance
- Low pulmonary vascular resistance

6. Cardiovascular examination (II): jugular venous pressure (JVP)

Questions

This is Mr Smith – you have been called to see him on the ward as he is acutely short of breath. As part of your general examination you examine his JVP. Please demonstrate how you would do this.

a) How will you position the patient for this examination? (2 marks)
b) How high should the jugular venous pressure (JVP) wave extend above the sternal angle in a healthy individual in this position when sitting up? (2 marks)
c) How can you exaggerate the JVP? (1 mark)
d) How do you distinguish the carotid pulse from the JVP? (6 marks)
e) What are the components of the JVP and what do they represent in the cardiac cycle? (5 marks)
f) When might you expect the JVP to be raised? (4 marks)

Answers

a) How will you position the patient for this examination? (2 marks)
- At a 45° recline
- Ask the patient to turn their head to the left, and ensure their neck muscles are relaxed by providing a pillow

b) How high should the JVP wave extend above the sternal angle in a healthy individual in this position when sitting up? (2 marks)
- No further than 4cm vertically from the sternal angle when the patient is semi recumbent at 45°
- Not visible when sitting

This is because in Man right atrial pressure is <7mmHg (9cmH$_2$0). The sternal angle is approximately 5cm above the right atrium. Therefore, the JVP should not extend more than 4cm above the sternal angle. In a healthy individual sitting upright the JVP should be hidden behind the clavicles.

c) How can you exaggerate the JVP? (1 mark)
- Hepatojugular reflex. Pressure on the liver causes 'back pressure' in the column of venous blood and so the JVP will rise

d) How do you distinguish the carotid pulse from the JVP? (6 marks)
- The carotid pulse is palpable, it is independent of position, and there is only one peak per heartbeat
- This is in contrast to the JVP, which is impalpable, dependent on position, diminished by pressure at the root of the neck, normally falls on inspiration, and has two peaks per heartbeat
- The JVP fills from above and can therefore be occluded from above

e) What are the components of the JVP and what do they represent in the cardiac cycle? (5 marks)
- The 'a' wave is the first peak. It coincides with atrial contraction and occurs just before the first heart sound
- The second peak, or the 'v' wave is due to atrial filling during ventricular systole whilst the tricuspid valve is closed
- The x descent occurs between the 'a' wave and the 'v' wave, and is due to fall in atrial pressure during ventricular systole
- The y descent occurs following the 'v' wave, and is due to opening of the tricuspid valve and passive filling of the ventricles
- A third peak, the 'c' wave is due to closure of the tricuspid valve and occurs during the x descent

f) When might you expect the JVP to be raised? (4 marks)
- Cardiac failure
- Fluid overload (e.g. renal failure, hepatic failure and IV fluid administration)
- Mechanical obstruction of the superior vena cava
- Massive pulmonary embolus, pericardial effusion or pericardial constriction

7. Cardiovascular examination (III): blood pressure and pulse

Questions

Please examine this patient's cardiovascular system.

a) How will you begin this examination? (3 marks)
b) How will you examine the pulse and what would you comment on? (6 marks)
c) What stage of the examination will you proceed to next? (2 marks)
d) What specifications for the equipment do you require and why? (2 marks)
e) How do you use the sphygmomanometer and what are the Korotkoff sounds? (4 marks)
f) How will you examine the precordium? (3 marks)

Answers

a) How will you begin this examination? (3 marks)
- Always begin your examination stations by introducing yourself to the patient
- Briefly explain what you are about to do
- Comment on their general appearance and clinical condition

b) How will you examine the pulse and what would you comment on? (6 marks)

You should examine both a peripheral pulse (usually the radial pulse), and a central pulse such as the carotid, for:
- Rate and Rhythm: In the exam the patient is likely to be in sinus rhythm between 60–100bpm, although they may have a physiological bradycardia. It is unlikely (but not impossible) that the patient may have atrial fibrillation or atrial ectopics; it is more likely they would have a sinus arrhythmia. To distinguish between these rhythms you would need an ECG
- Volume: volume of the pulse reflects the pulse pressure, that is the difference between systolic and diastolic pressures
- Character: a slow rising pulse is characteristic of aortic stenosis, whereas a collapsing pulse is characteristic of aortic regurgitation

A large volume pulse may be due to aortic regurgitation or a high output state such as pregnancy, exercise, emotion and heat. A low volume pulse may be due to heart failure or peripheral vascular disease, a 'weak and thready' pulse occurs in hypovolaemia. A bounding pulse can be caused by CO_2 retention, liver failure and sepsis.

c) What stage of the examination will you proceed to next? (2 marks)
- Measure the patient's blood pressure using a manual sphygmomanometer

d) What specifications for the equipment do you require and why? (2 marks)
- A bladder length of 30–35cm and a width of 12cm (40% of arm circumference)
- A cuff that is too small will give an elevated reading and vice versa

e) How do you use the sphygmomanometer and what are the Korotkoff sounds? (4 marks)
- Inflate the cuff until the radial pulse is impalpable, and then deflate and repeat with the stethoscope placed over the brachial artery. Reinflate to 10mmHg above the previous systolic reading
- This time, on deflating the cuff you can listen for the re-emergence of the first Korotkoff sound which indicates the systolic BP and then the muffling or disappearance of sounds (4th or 5th Korotkoff sounds) which will indicate the diastolic blood pressure. Traditionally the 4th sound (muffling) was used to estimate diastolic pressure but more recently the 5th sound (start of silence) has been adopted, as it is more reproducible. In paediatrics the 5th sound is used but in pregnancy often the 4th sound is quoted as more accurate

f) How will you examine the precordium? (3 marks)
- **Inspection**
- **Palpation**
- **Auscultation**

Inspect: For surgical scars (midline sternotomy or thoracotomy), visible pulsations (heaves), and chest deformity.
Palpate: For the apex beat (you may ask the patient to lie to their left), and for thrills (palpable murmurs).

Auscultate: Initially listening for the 1st and 2nd heart sound, and additional sounds. The third heart sound is due to rapid filling of the ventricles and may be normal in children, young adults and during pregnancy, but also occurs in left ventricular failure and mitral regurgitation. The fourth heart sound is *always* pathological and is due to an atrial contraction against a non-compliant ventricle such as in ventricular hypertrophy, hypertension and aortic stenosis. It is best heard with the bell at the apex. Then listen for further sounds such as the metallic click of a replaced heart valve. You should listen for murmurs at the aortic, pulmonary, tricuspid and apical regions. You should also listen for radiation at the carotids.

8. Respiratory examination

Questions

Mr Clarke has attended for a transurethral resection of prostate (TURP). He is on domicilary oxygen for his chronic obstructive pulmonary disease (COPD). Please examine him and then interpret the test results.

a) What positive signs may you observe from the end of the bed? (5 marks)

b) What might you see on examination of his hands? (3 marks)

c) What may you expect to find on examination of the chest? (4 marks)

d) What common tests could you be asked to interpret and what might they show in a patient with COPD? (4 marks)

e) What considerations will you be making for anaesthetic care? (4 marks)

Answers

a) What positive signs may you observe from the end of the bed? (5 marks)
- Poor general condition and cachexia
- Use of accessory muscles of respiration
- Respiratory Rate
- Cyanosis
- Hyperexpansion of the chest

b) What might you see on examination of his hands? (3 marks)
- Clubbing (from co-existing suppurative lung condition)
- Peripheral cyanosis
- Nicotine staining

c) What may you expect to find on examination of the chest? (4 marks)
- Inspection: Hyperexpansion, scars or other skeletal deformities
- Palpation: is there equal expansion?
- Percussion: hyperresonance (due to gas trapping or massive bullae) or dullness (due to consolidation or effusion)
- Auscultation: breath sounds may be reduced or you may detect early inspiratory crackles.
- Perform a test for vocal resonance

d) What common tests could you be asked to interpret and what might they show in a patient with COPD? (4 marks)
- Baseline arterial blood gas
  - This may show type I or type II respiratory failure. This is helpful in targeting intra-operative and postoperative oxygen saturations, predicting tolerance of oxygen therapy and reliance of hypoxia on respiratory drive. A resting pCO_2 of >6kPa is predictive of pulmonary complications
- Spirometry
  - You may be presented with spirometry results. In COPD there is an obstructive deficit so the forced vital capacity (FVC) may be normal but the FEV1 will be markedly reduced. The FEV1/FVC will be <75% (normal value 75–80%). A FEV1 <1L is predictive of post-operative complications due to poor cough and secretion clearance. This may indicate the need for increased respiratory support post operatively

e) What considerations will you be making for anaesthetic care? (4 marks)
- Consider regional anaesthetic techniques
- Consider HDU/ICU post-operatively
- Early nebulisers
- Early physiotherapy
- Seek input from respiratory physicians

9. Examination of a patient following a head injury

Questions

You are asked to assess Mr Beasley who has suffered a head injury. He is already in a collar and blocks and his airway has been cleared during the primary survey.

a) What sort of head injuries are commonly seen in trauma patients? (4 marks)

b) How do start your examination? (1 mark)

c) How do you assess the patient's conscious level? (4 marks)

d) What will you be looking for on examining the pupils? (1 mark)

e) How will you complete your examination? (3 marks)

f) What are the indications for immediate intubation and ventilation following a head injury? (3 marks)

g) What considerations should be made on induction of anaesthesia? (2 marks)

h) What is the Cushing Response? (1 mark)

Answers

a) What sort of head injuries are commonly seen in trauma patients? (4 marks)

Any 4 out of:
- Focal scalp injury
- Depressed vault fracture
- Extradural haemorrhage
- Focal brain injury
- Contra-coup injury
- Brain laceration and intracranial haemorrhage
- Subdural haemorrhage

b) How do start your examination? (1 mark)
- You will need to start by introducing yourself and explaining to the patient what you are going to do

c) How do you assess the patient's conscious level? (4 marks)
- Formally examine the level of consciousness using the Glasgow Coma Scale. Level of consciousness is the main indicator of global brain function

Table 5.1 Glasgow Coma Scale

Response Elicited	Score
Response of Eyes	
Opens Spontaneously	4
Opens to Voice	3
Opens to Pain	2
Does not Open	1
Best Motor Response	
Obeys Commands	6
Localises to Pain	5
Withdraws from Pain	4
Flexes to Pain (de-corticate response)	3
Extends to Pain (de-cerebrate response)	2
No response	1
Best Verbal Response	
Orientated	5
Confused	4
Inappropriate words	3
Incomprehensible sounds	2
No verbal response	1

Reprinted from *The Lancet*, 304, Teasdale G and Jennett B, Assessment of coma and impaired consciousness: a practical scale, 81–4. Copyright (1974) with permission from Elsevier

A decreased level of consciousness may indicate intracranial pathology if other causes such as hypoxia, hypothermia, hypoglycaemia, toxins or gross metabolic disturbances have been ruled out.

d) What will you be looking for on examining the pupils? (1 mark)

- Size
- Reactivity (direct and consensual) to light

It is important to examine the pupils for size and reactivity. Unilateral or bilateral 'blown pupils' (pupils that are increased in size and unreactive to light) are indicative of ipsilateral intracranial pathology and raised intracranial pressure. In a patient with a decreased conscious level of unknown cause it is important to consider opiate narcosis and characteristic 'pinpoint pupils'.

e) How will you complete your examination? (3 marks)

- Examine the scalp for lacerations, swellings and crepitus
- Examine auditory canals and tympanic membranes
- A full neurological examination for focal neurological deficits should be carried out

f) What are the indications for immediate intubation and ventilation following a head injury? (3 marks)

- Coma or deteriorating conscious level
- Loss of protective airway reflexes
- Ventilatory failure (aim for a PaO_2 of >13kPa and a pCO_2 of 4.5–5kPa)
- Multiple seizures
- Significant facial injuries
- Bleeding into the airway

g) What considerations should be made on induction of anaesthesia? (2 marks)

- C-spine precautions should be taken, and manual inline stabilisation maintained
- Suppression of the laryngeal response to prevent an increase in intracranial pressure
- Maintain cerebral perfusion pressure throughout induction, aiming for a mean arterial pressure (MAP)>80 This may require vasopressor support

h) What is the Cushing Response? (1 mark)

- The Cushing Response is a late and often terminal sign of raised intracranial pressure and herniation of the brain through the foramen magnum. It is the combination of bradycardia and hypertension in the context of dilated and unreactive pupils

Further reading

Douglas G, Nicol F, Robertson C. *Macleods Clinical Examination* (13th edn). Churchill Livingstone, 2013

Chapter 6 **Radiology**

Introduction

There will be two radiology stations in your OSCE. Traditionally these tested the ability to interpret chest X-rays but in recent years these stations have included CT and MRI scans. Often, very few marks are awarded for interpretation of the image and it is used as a stem to test broader knowledge of that topic.

Questions are usually 'true or false' questions.

1. Chest X-ray Case 1

Questions

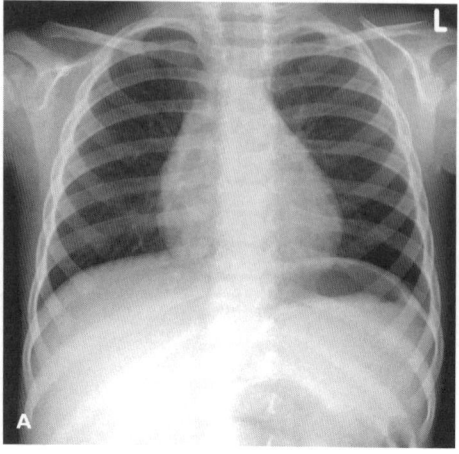 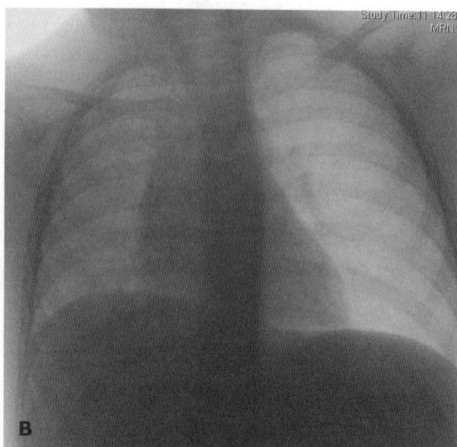

Figure 6.1a Chest X-ray   **Figure 6.1b** Chest X-ray

a) Look at Figure 6.1a. Adequate inspiration was achieved when this chest X-ray (CXR) was taken. (1 mark)

b) This is a paediatric film. (1 mark)

c) There is consolidation on the right side. (1 mark)

d) Figure 6.1b is an expiratory film. (1 mark)

e) This CXR could be consistent with an inhaled foreign body. (1 mark)

f) Right lower lobar collapse can cause mediastinal shift. (1 mark)

g) Inspiratory and expiratory films are useful in cases of inhaled foreign bodies when there is collapse. (I mark)

h) The 3rd generation of the bronchial tree is the most common place for foreign bodies to lodge. (1 mark)

i) It is advantageous to preserve spontaneous ventilation during bronchoscopic removal of a foreign body. (1 mark)

j) The most likely cause of an intraoperative bradycardia during removal of a foreign body would be a pneumothorax. (1 mark)

Answers

a) Look at Figure 6.1a. Adequate inspiration was achieved when this CXR was taken. (1 mark)
- True

    Chest X-rays are usually taken during the inspiratory phase to allow maximum visualization of the lung bases. When the diaphragm is intersected by the 5th–7th ribs in the midclavicular line the patient has performed adequate inspiration.

b) This is a paediatric film. (1 mark)
- True

    This is an X-ray of a 2-year-old. In paediatric films the thymus maybe visible as a mediastinal mass and the costophrenic angles may be shallower.

c) There is consolidation on the right side. (1 mark)
- False

    There is gas trapping on the left side which makes it appear more radiolucent than the right.

d) Figure 6.1b is an expiratory film. (1 mark)
- True

    Usually chest films are taken during inspiration. To aid the diagnosis of an inhaled foreign body, often expiratory films are requested as gas trapping maybe seen more clearly. In this X-ray only the 4th rib intersects the diaphragm on the right; this should usually be the 5th–7th rib in an inspiratory film.

e) This CXR could be consistent with an inhaled foreign body. (1 mark)
- True

    The foreign body may not be visualized particularly if it is made of organic matter. Beyond the obstruction, gas trapping (seen here), collapse or consolidation can occur.

f) Right lower lobar collapse can cause mediastinal shift. (1 mark)
- True

    Collapse of any lobe can cause mediastinal shift or a change in position of a hemidiaphragm.

g) Inspiratory and expiratory films are useful in cases of inhaled foreign bodies when there is collapse. (1 mark)
- True

    Lobar collapse may not be seen during inspiration as the diameter of the airways is larger, however, during expiration collapse can occur and is highly suggestive of an obstruction of the larger airways.

h) The 3rd generation of the bronchial tree is the most common place for foreign bodies to lodge. (1 mark)
- False

    90% of foreign bodies lodge in the main bronchi.

i) It is advantageous to preserve spontaneous ventilation during bronchoscopic removal of a foreign body. (1 mark)
- True

    Positive pressure ventilation may increase air trapping and cause a pneumothorax and may also force the foreign body further down the bronchial tree.

j) The most likely cause of an intraoperative bradycardia during removal of a foreign body would be a pneumothorax. (1 mark)
- False

    The most common cause of bradycardia would be hypoxia.

2. Chest X-ray Case 2

Questions

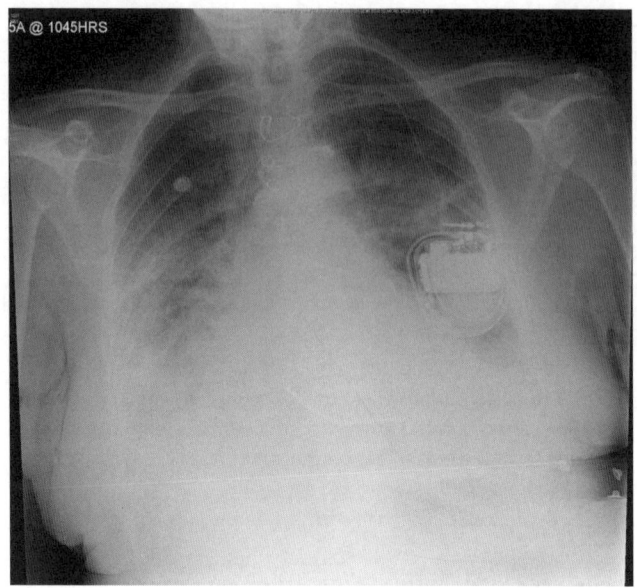

Figure 6.2 X-ray Case 2

Look at Figure 6.2

a) This is a PA (posteroior – anterior) film. (1 mark)

b) This patient has cardiomegaly. (1 mark)

c) This patient is expected to have a high pulmonary capillary wedge pressure. (1 mark)

d) The internal device is implantable defibrillator. (1 mark)

e) Unipolar diathermy is preferable in this patient as long as they are fully monitored. (1 mark)

f) The leads of the device are intact. (1 mark)

g) Use of a magnet will usually prevent the implantable cardioverter-defibrillator (ICD) defibrillating function even after it is removed. (1 mark)

h) This patient has pulmonary oedema. (1 mark)

i) The most likely diagnosis is acute respiratory distress syndrome (ARDS). (1 mark)

j) Pleural effusions in cardiac failure are always bilateral. (1 mark)

Answers

Look at Figure 6.2

a) This is a PA (posteroior – anterior) film. (1 mark)
- False

This is an AP (anterior-posterior film). Unless stated otherwise films are usually taken in the PA position (i.e. with the patient facing away from the radiation source, towards the screen). Sick patients may well have X-rays in the AP position as they may be shot from above on an emergency department trolley or in bed. PA films can be identified as the medial borders of the scapulae are usually retracted laterally and the cardiac shadow is smaller.

b) This patient has cardiomegaly. (1 mark)
- True

Although this is an AP film, so the heart size is less accurate, it is clearly enlarged. A cardio-thoracic ratio of >50% (on a PA film) is suggestive of enlarged heart size.

c) This patient is expected to have a high pulmonary capillary wedge pressure. (1 mark)
- True

This patient has cardiomegaly, upper lobe blood diversion and pulmonary oedema in keeping with severe congestive cardiac failure. Therefore, their pulmonary capillary wedge pressures are likely to be high. Interstitial oedema occurs with pressures between 18–25mm Hg and alveolar oedema with pressures greater than 25mm Hg.

d) The internal device is implantable defibrillator. (1 mark)
- True

ICDs usually have one or both leads that are wider than a pacemaker lead. An ICD lead should terminate in the right ventricle.

e) Unipolar diathermy is preferable in this patient as long as they are fully monitored. (1 mark)
- False

Bipolar diathermy is preferable in patients with ICDs to reduce the risk of interference and unnecessary discharge.

f) The leads of the device are intact. (1 mark)
- True

There are no obvious fractures in the lead.

g) Use of a magnet will usually prevent the ICD defibrillating function even after it is removed. (1 mark)
- False

Usually the defibrillator function is only impaired whilst in contact with the magnet. Most modern ICDs will revert back to their normal function once the magnet has been removed although a thorough test of the device by a cardiac technician is recommended after exposure to a magnet.

h) This patient has pulmonary oedema. (1 mark)
- True

The patient has bilateral pleural effusions and peri-hilar interstitial shadowing in keeping with pulmonary oedema.

i) The most likely diagnosis is ARDS. (1 mark)
- False

Although pulmonary oedema is a sign of ARDS, this patient has cardiomegaly and upper lobe blood diversion making cardiac failure the most likely diagnosis.

j) Pleural effusions in cardiac failure are always bilateral. (1 mark)
- False

Effusions are bilateral in 70% of patients with congestive cardiac failure.

3. Chest X-ray Case 3

Questions

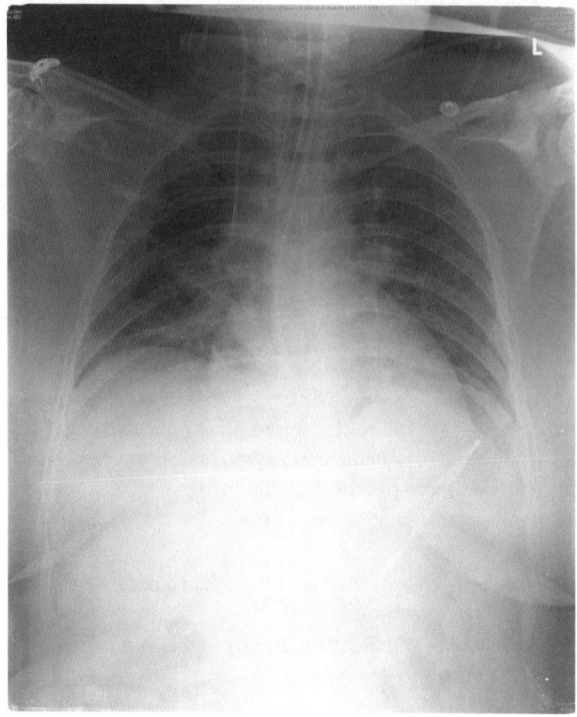

Figure 6.3 Chest X-ray

Look at Figure 6.3

a) This CXR is rotated. (1 mark)

b) The endo-tracheal tube is optimally positioned. (1 mark)

c) In an adult, the tip of an endotracheal tube moves by 0.5cm on flexion of the neck. (1 mark)

d) The patient is likely to have fever and a high white cell count. (1 mark)

e) The trachea is deviated. (1 mark)

f) This patient is at risk of developing a tension pneumothorax. (1 mark)

g) The left upper lobe bronchus arises closer to the carina than the right. (1 mark)

h) The carina lies at the level of the T6 vertebral body in an adult. (1 mark)

i) There would be decreased air entry on the left of the patient's chest. (1 mark)

j) The patient requires re-intubation. (1 mark)

Answers

Look at Figure 6.3

a) This CXR is rotated. (1 mark)
  - False

    The spinous processes of the vertebrae are in the midline and are equidistant from the medial ends of the clavicles.

b) The endo-tracheal tube is optimally positioned. (1 mark)
  - False

    The tube tip is in the right main bronchus.

c) In an adult, the tip of an endotracheal tube moves by 0.5cm on flexion of the neck. (1 mark)
  - False

    The tip of an endotracheal tube has been shown to move by up to 2cm with flexion of the neck.

d) The patient is likely to have fever and a high white cell count. (1 mark)
  - False

    When right-sided endobronchial intubation occurs you may see right upper lobe collapse and poor inflation of the left lung (not visible in this image). It can be difficult to differentiate between collapse and consolidation but the position of the tube means that collapse will be more likely as a result of an obstruction of the upper 2nd generation bronchus leading to the upper lobe.

e) The trachea is deviated. (1 mark)
  - False

    The trachea is in the midline.

f) This patient is at risk of developing a tension pneumothorax. (1 mark)
  - True

    Endobronchial intubation can lead to high inflation pressures putting the patient at risk of a pneumothorax. This can become a tension pneumothorax and cause a life-threatening emergency.

g) The left upper lobe bronchus arises closer to the carina than the right. (1 mark)
  - False

    The origin of the right upper lobe bronchus is closer to the carina than the left putting it at greater risk of obstruction by endobronchial intubation or malpositioned double lumen tubes.

h) The carina lies at the level of the T6 vertebral body in an adult. (1 mark)
  - False

    The carina is at the level of T4.

i) There would be decreased air entry on the left of the patient's chest. (1 mark)
  - True

    Auscultation of the chest would reveal decreased air entry on the left as a result of right-sided endobronchial intubation, although transmitted breath sounds may be heard.

j) The patient requires re-intubation. (1 mark)
  - False

    The tube needs to be repositioned, i.e. withdrawn into the trachea, but re-intubation is not necessarily required. Confirmation of its placement should be sought after any manipulation.

4. Lateral chest X-ray

Questions

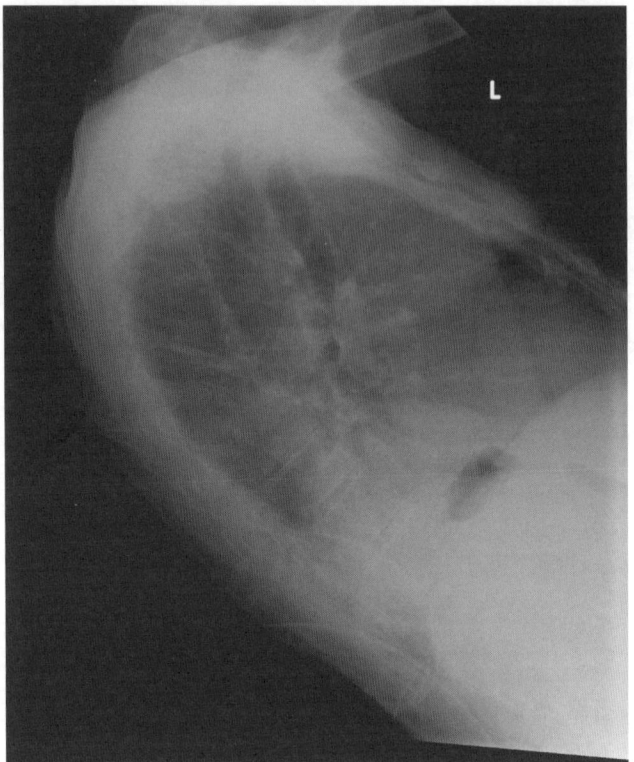

Figure 6.4 Lateral chest X-ray

Look at Figure 6.4

a) Radiolucency of the retrosternal space is pathological. (1 mark)

b) In a lateral film, the vertebral bodies may become more radiolucent as they proceed caudally. (1 mark)

c) This patient has a pneumothorax. (1 mark)

d) A rapid sequence induction should be performed on this patient. (1 mark)

e) The middle mediastinum contains the oesophagus. (1 mark)

f) A lateral CXR requires less radiation exposure than a PA chest film. (1 mark)

g) This patient's abdominal condition would not be visible on a PA chest X-ray. (1 mark)

h) Aspiration pneumonitis should always be treated with antibiotics. (1 mark)

i) The mortality associated with aspiration pneumonia in symptomatic patients is 50%. (1 mark)

j) Low pH gastric contents are more harmful than those with a higher pH. (1 mark)

Answers

Look at Figure 6.4

a) Radiolucency of the retrosternal space is pathological. (1 mark)
- False

  The retrosternal space is normally radiolucent. Any opacity would be suggestive of an anterior mediastinal mass.

b) In a lateral film, the vertebral bodies may become more radiolucent as they proceed caudally. (1 mark)
- True

  Less dense overlying tissue is present in the inferior thorax compared with the superior.

c) This patient has a pneumothorax. (1 mark)
- False

  The radiolucent area is a hiatus hernia.

d) A rapid sequence induction should be performed on this patient. (1 mark)
- True

  This patient has a significant hiatus hernia and is at risk of aspiration on induction.

e) The middle mediastinum contains the oesophagus. (1 mark)
- True

  The middle mediastinal compartment contains the oesophagus, vena cava, azygous vein, aortic arch, lymph nodes, trachea and posterior heart.

f) A lateral CXR requires less radiation exposure than a PA chest film. (1 mark)
- False

  The lateral CXR is associated with higher radiation (0.05 vs 0.02 mSv).

g) This patient's abdominal condition would not be visible on a PA chest X-ray. (1 mark)
- False

  A hiatus hernia may be seen as a fluid level in the thorax on an PA film or a gas shadow seen through the cardiac shadow.

h) Aspiration pneumonitis should always be treated with antibiotics. (1 mark)
- False

  Antibiotics should not be prescribed unless there is evidence of an aspiration **pneumonia.**

i) The mortality associated with aspiration pneumonia in symptomatic patients is 50%. (1 mark)
- False

  In patients who have aspirated, about two thirds will not develop symptoms. In those that develop symptoms, mortality remains high at about 10%.

j) Low pH gastric contents are more harmful than those with a higher pH (1 mark)
- True

  The severity of the lung injury increases as pH decreases and as volume of aspirate increases.

5. C-spine X-ray Case 1

Questions

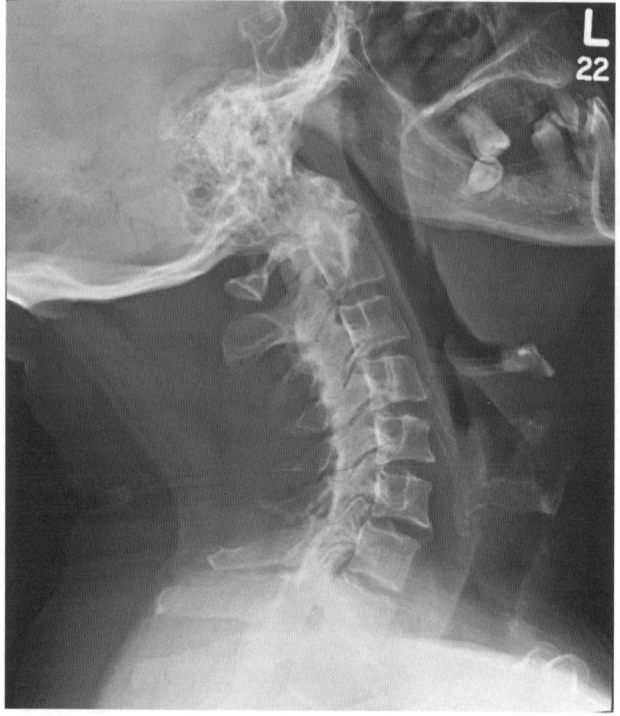

Figure 6.5 C-spine X-ray

Look at Figure 6.5

a) The view of this lateral c-spine is adequate. (1 mark)

b) Alignment is assessed due to the continuity of the curve along 4 lines. (1 mark)

c) A fracture can be seen in the C4 vertebrae. (1 mark)

d) There is evidence of rheumatoid disease. (1 mark)

e) All patients who have antlanto-axial subluxation (AAS) as a result of rheumatoid disease will have neurological signs and symptoms. (1 mark)

f) The most common form of AAS is anterior movement of C1 on C2. (1 mark)

g) Patients with rheumatoid arthritis may have a hoarse voice. (1 mark)

h) This patient should be managed with manual in-line stabilisation for intubation. (1 mark)

i) Mouth opening may be impaired in this patient. (1 mark)

j) You should consider steroid supplementation. (1 mark)

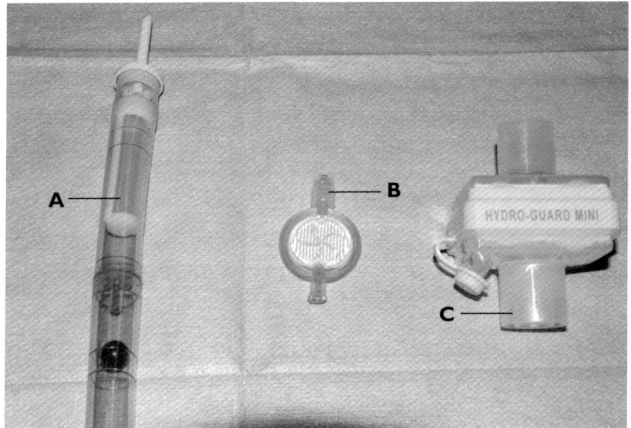

Figure 7.1 Filters

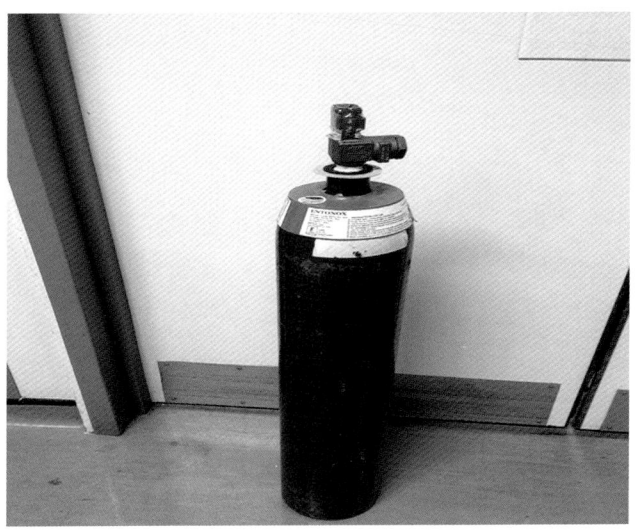

Figure 7.2 Cylinder

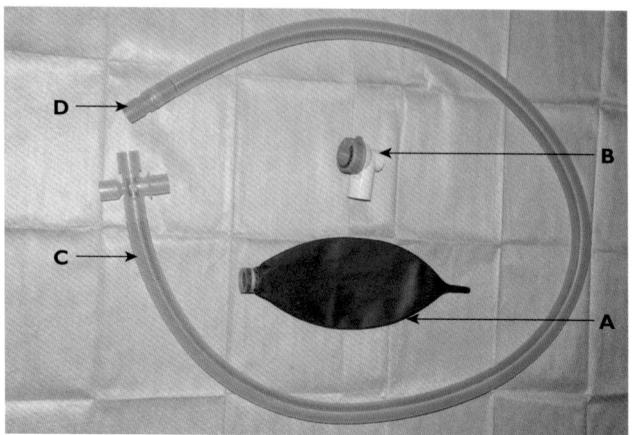

Figure 7.3 Circuit components

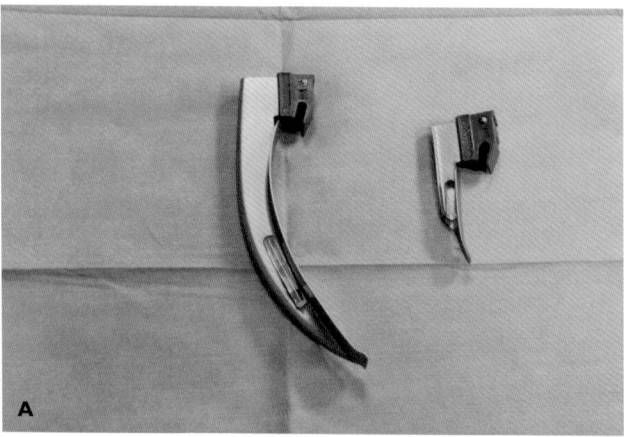

Figure 7.4a Laryngoscopes

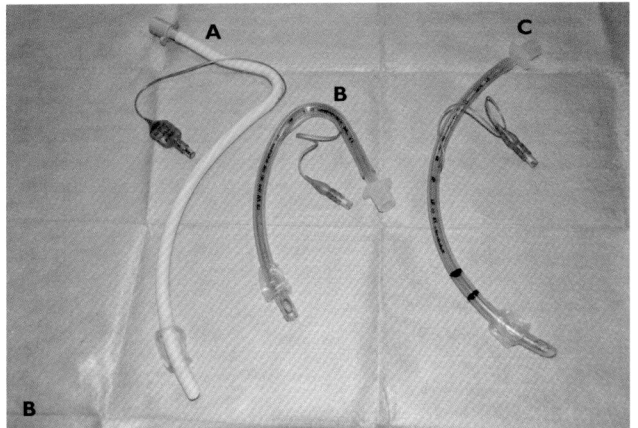

Figure 7.4b Tubes

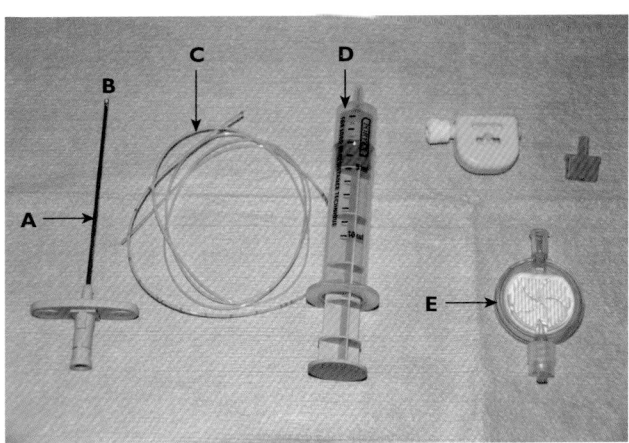

Figure 7.5 Epidurals

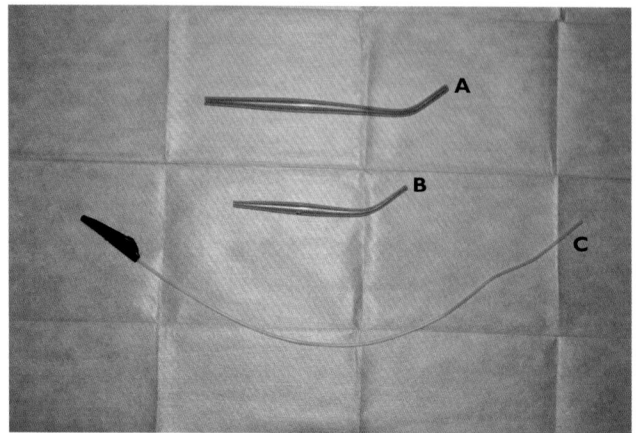

Figure 7.6 Suction

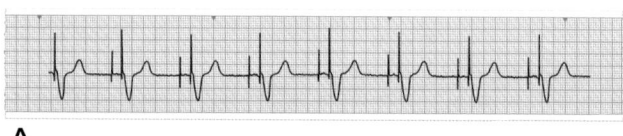

Figure 7.7a ECG

ECG, Courtesy of Dr Oliver Meyer

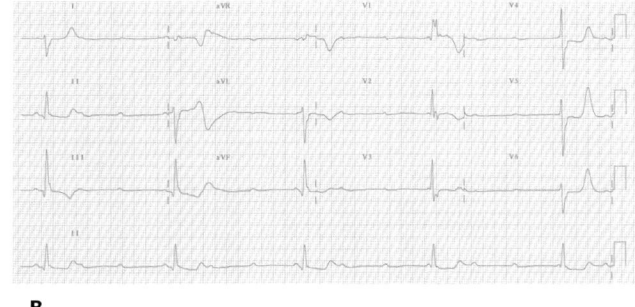

B

Figure 7.7b ECG

Reproduced from Myerson SG et al., *Emergencies in Cardiology*, 2009 with permission from Oxford University Press

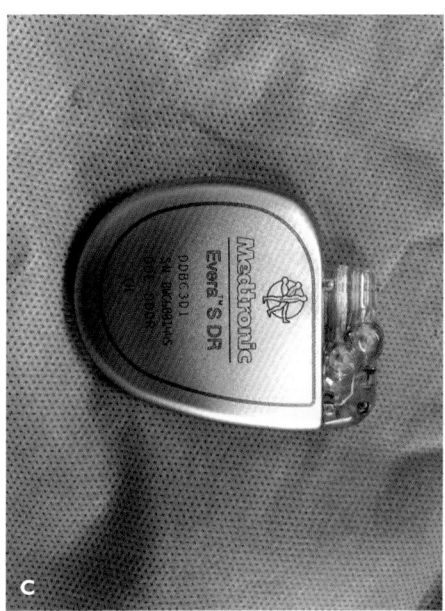

Figure 7.7c Defibrillator

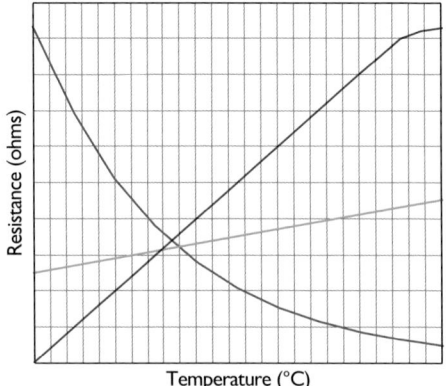

Figure 9.1 Graph

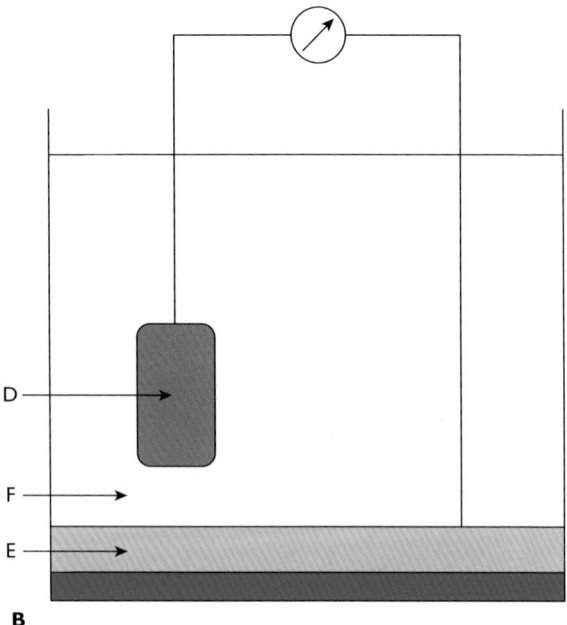

Figure 9.5b Fuel cell

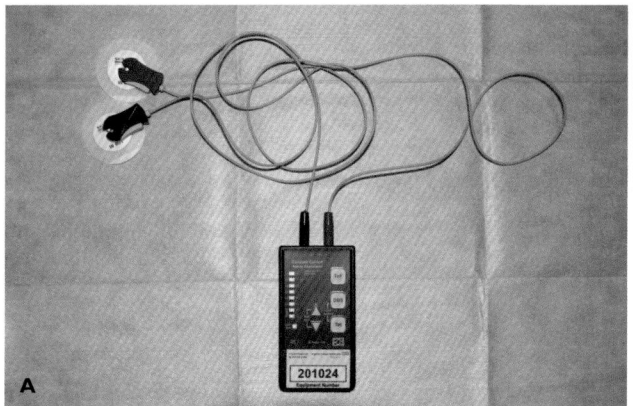

Figure 9.6a Equipment to stimulate nerves

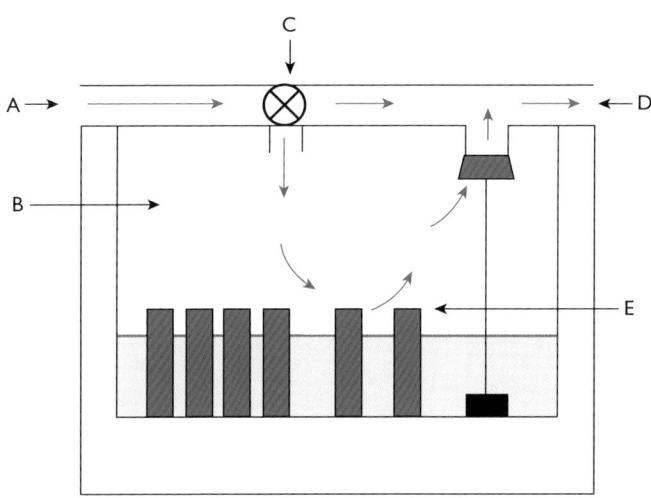

Figure 9.7 Vaporiser

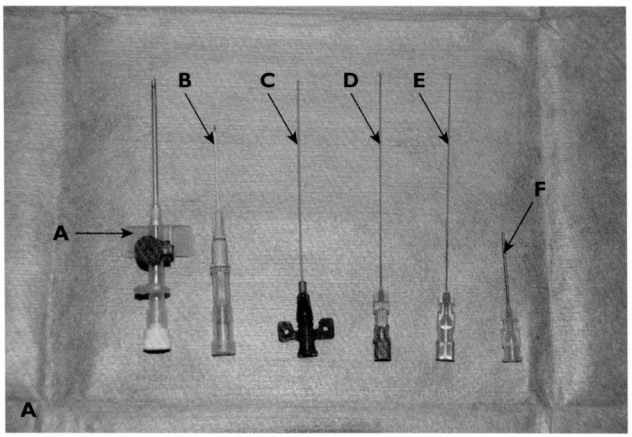

Figure 11.3a Needles and cannulas

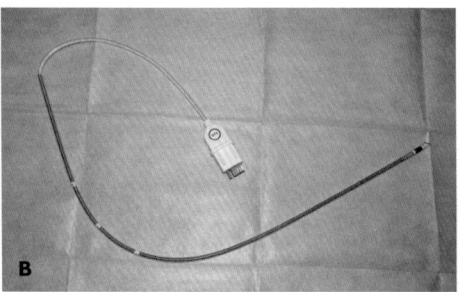

Figure 11.4b Probe

Answers

Look at Figure 6.5

a) The view of this lateral c-spine is adequate. (1 mark)
- True
  The lateral view of the cervical spine must show the C7/T1 disc space.

b) Alignment is assessed due to the continuity of the curve along 4 lines. (1 mark)
- True
  There are 4 lines on a lateral c-spine X-ray that, if continuous, confirm correct alignment. 'Steps' in these lines can indicate a dislocation or subluxation. Normal slight lordosis is lost in severe muscle spasm. The 4 lines are as follows:
  - Anterior borders of the vertebral bodies
  - Posterior borders of the vertebral bodies (anterior boundary of the vertebral canal)
  - Posterior boundary of the vertebral canal
  - Tips of the spinous processes

c) A fracture can be seen in the C4 vertebrae. (1 mark)
- False
  The height and shape of each vertebral body should be compared for wedging and fractures. Facets and spinous processes should also be examined. Soft tissue shadowing, anterior to the vertebral bodies, is increased if there is a fracture, haematoma or anterior ligament injury. Above the larynx the width of the prevertebral soft tissue space should be less than one third of the diameter of the vertebral body. Below this level the space is accepted as normal if it is no wider than a whole vertebral body.

d) There is evidence of rheumatoid disease. (1 mark)
- True
  There is severe erosive disease of the dens.

e) All patients who have AAS as a result of rheumatoid disease will have neurological signs and symptoms. (1 mark)
- False
  AAS occurs in 25% of patients with rheumatoid arthritis, only 25% of these patients will have neurological signs and symptoms.

f) The most common form of AAS is anterior movement of C1 on C2. (1 mark)
- True
  80% of AAS in rheumatoid arthritis is due to anterior AAS where you will see C1 forward on C2 from destruction of the transverse ligament. It is significant if there is a gap of >3mm between the ondontoid and the arch of the atlas in lateral flexion radiographs.

g) Patients with rheumatoid arthritis may have a hoarse voice. (1 mark)
- True
  Rheumatoid involvement of the cricoarytenoid joints may lead to voice changes, hoarseness, and rarely to stridor from glottic stenosis. In this situation an ENT opinion should be sought and nasendoscopy performed.

h) This patient should be managed with manual in-line stabilisation for intubation. (1 mark)
- False
  The patient should be assessed clinically and further radiology requested. Instability from the dens erosion may mean that this patient requires stabilisation surgery prior to other elective surgery. In an emergency manual in-line stabilisation may be adequate, but awake fibreoptic intubation would be more appropriate in both emergency and elective situations.

i) Mouth opening may be impaired in this patient. (1 mark)

- True

  Temporomandibular joint stiffness can occur with rheumatoid arthritis, further complicating intubation.

j) You should consider steroid supplementation. (1 mark)

- True

  You should consider steroid supplementation if the patient is taking over 10mg of prednisolone per day or if they have had a recent course (past 3 months) of high dose steroids.

6. C-spine X-ray Case 2

Questions

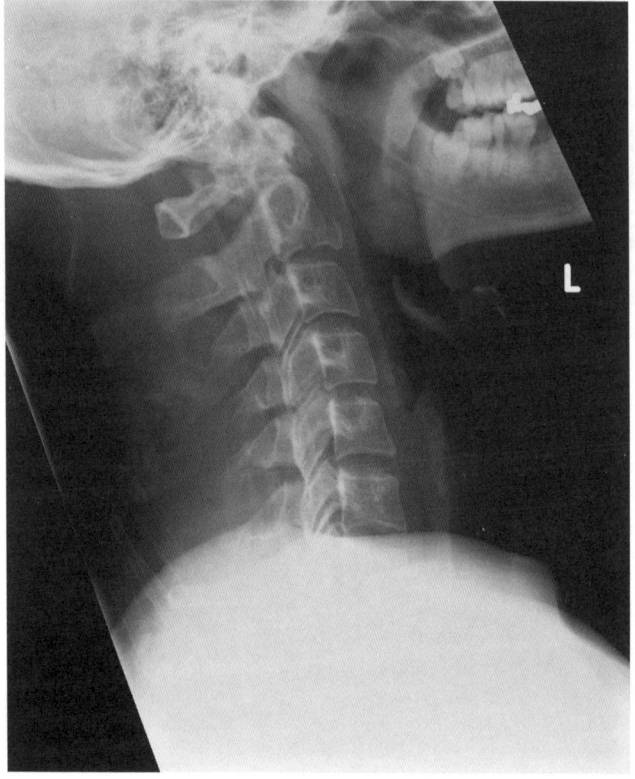

Figure 6.6 C-spine X-ray Case 2

Look at Figure 6.6

a) This demonstrates a fracture of the ondontoid peg of C2 (the axis). (1 mark)

b) If this patient presents with pins-and-needles in their fingers following a RTA they need immediate intubation. (1 mark)

c) This injury is typically due to excessive flexion. (1 mark)

d) C2 is the most common cervical vertebra to be fractured in adults. (1 mark)

e) The most common C1 fracture is a burst fracture. (Jefferson fracture). (1 mark)

f) The Jefferson fracture is usually a stable fracture. (1 mark)

g) 5% of patients with a brain injury have an associated spinal injury. (1 mark)

h) Approximately one-third of patients with an upper cervical cord injury die at the scene of the accident. (1 mark)

i) Spinal cord injury at C6 will not have an effect on ventilation. (1 mark)

j) Neurogenic shock occurs with lesions above T6. (1 mark)

Answers

Look at Figure 6.6

a) This demonstrates a fracture of the ondontoid peg of C2 (the axis). (1 mark)
- False

   This demonstrates an anterior plate 'teardrop' fracture of C2. Other traumatic fractures include the 'Hangman's' fracture: a fracture of the posterior elements of C2 – the pars interarticularis.

b) If this patient presents with pins-and-needles in their fingers following a RTA they need immediate intubation. (1 mark)
- False

   This patient requires immobilisation on a spinal board and semi-rigid collar and immediate orthopaedic input. The patient should be intubated if there is evidence of respiratory compromise.

c) This injury is typically due to excessive flexion. (1 mark)
- True

   This is usually caused by excessive flexion. A 'Hangman's' fracture is typically due to extension.

d) C2 is the most common cervical vertebra to be fractured in adults. (1 mark)
- False

   C5 is the most commonly fractured cervical vertebra and C3 is the least commonly fractured.

e) The most common C1 fracture is a burst fracture (Jefferson fracture). (1 mark)
- True

   The usual mechanism is axial loading, due to a large load falling on the person's head, or the person falling vertically onto their head.

f) The Jefferson fracture is usually a stable fracture. (1 mark)
- False

   These fractures are not usually associated with spinal cord injuries (due to the width of the spinal canal at this level), but they are unstable fractures and require treatment with a cervical collar.

g) 5% of patients with a brain injury have an associated spinal injury. (1 mark)
- True

   55% of these occur in the cervical area.

h) Approximately one-third of patients with an upper cervical cord injury die at the scene of the accident. (I mark)
- True

i) Spinal cord injury at C6 will not have an effect on ventilation. (1 mark)
- False

   Despite diaphragmatic innervation arising from C3/4/5 nerve roots, an injury at C6 may cause damage to the innervation of intercostal and abdominal muscles meaning that expiration becomes entirely passive. This may also result in paradoxical chest wall movement and an inability to clear secretions adequately.

j) Neurogenic shock occurs with lesions above T6. (1 mark)
- True

   Lesions above T6 can result in the loss of sympathetic autonomic function with maintained, unopposed, parasympathetic innervation. The cardiac accelerator fibres may also be affected causing bradycardia in spite of the hypotension.

7. Lumbar spine X-ray

Questions

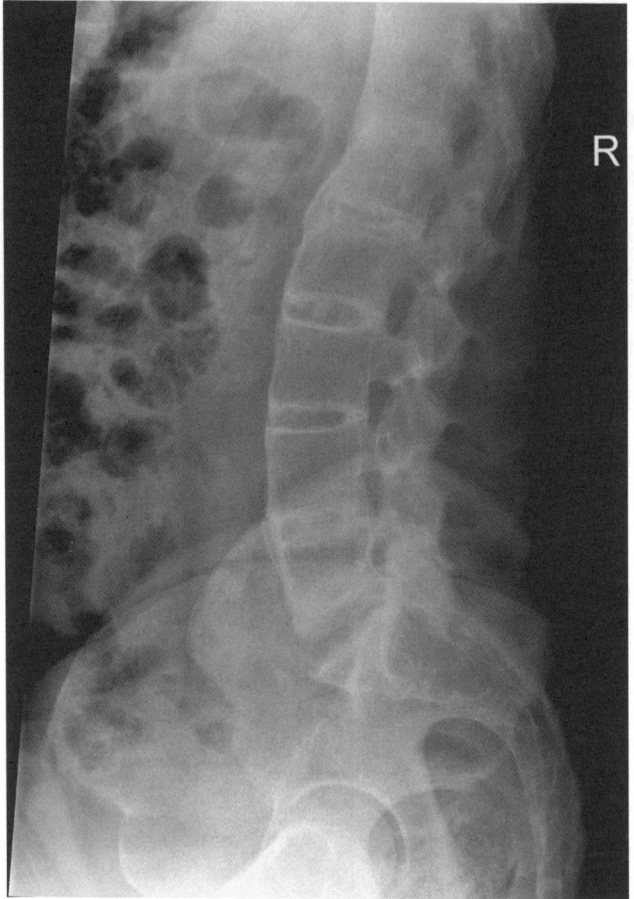

Figure 6.7 Lumbar spine X-ray

Look at Figure 6.7

a) This patient has osteoarthritis. (1 mark)
b) This patient may have limited mouth opening. (1 mark)
c) Pulmonary complications could occur post-operatively. (1 mark)
d) The female to male ratio of this condition is 4:1. (1 mark)
e) Neuroaxial block would be the ideal method of anaesthesia for this patient for total hip replacement. (1 mark)
f) Aortic stenosis is associated with this underlying condition. (1 mark)
g) You should stop any disease modifying agents in the peri-operative period. (1 mark)
h) You may find positioning this patient difficult. (1 mark)
i) In health the L4/5 disc space should be wider than the L5/S1 space. (1 mark)
j) Patients with this condition are at higher risk of complications from epidural insertion. (1 mark)

Answers

Look at Figure 6.7

a) This patient has osteoarthritis. (1 mark)
- False

This patient has the characteristic radiographic 'bamboo spine' appearance of ankolysing spondolysis.

b) This patient may have limited mouth opening. (1 mark)
- True

Temporomandibular joint involvement can limit mouth opening.

c) Pulmonary complications could occur post-operatively. (1 mark)
- True

  Patients with ankolysing spondolysis can have limited chest expansion due to skeletal deformities. In addition, these patients may have lung fibrosis (typically affecting the upper lobes), that can exacerbate post-operative hypoxia.

d) The female to male ratio of this condition is 4:1. (1 mark)
- False

  The male to female ratio of ankolysing spondolysis is 4:1.

e) Neuroaxial block would be the ideal method of anaesthesia for this patient for total hip replacement. (1 mark)
- False

  Axial skeletal involvement may make the neuroaxial approach difficult or even impossible. If required or preferred a paramedian approach may be the most practical technique.

f) Aortic stenosis is associated with this underlying condition. (1 mark)
- False

  There is a 1% incidence of aortic regurgitation in these patients.

g) You should stop any disease modifying agents in the peri-operative period. (1 mark)
- False

  You should continue all disease-modifying anti-rheumatic drugs (DMARDS) in the perioperative period as there is no evidence that omitting them reduces post-operative complications such as wound infection.

h) You may find positioning this patient difficult. (1 mark)
- True

  This is due to skeletal deformities and is particularly problematic for prone positioning.

i) In health the L4/5 disc space should be wider than the L5/S1 space. (1 mark)
- True

  Disc space gradually increases in height from superior to inferior, expect for L5/S1 which is usually slightly narrower than the L4/L5 space.

j) Patients with this condition are at higher risk of complications from epidural insertion. (1 mark)
- True

  There is an increased risk of spinal haematoma following epidural insertion in patients with ankylosing spondylitis.

8. CT head

Questions

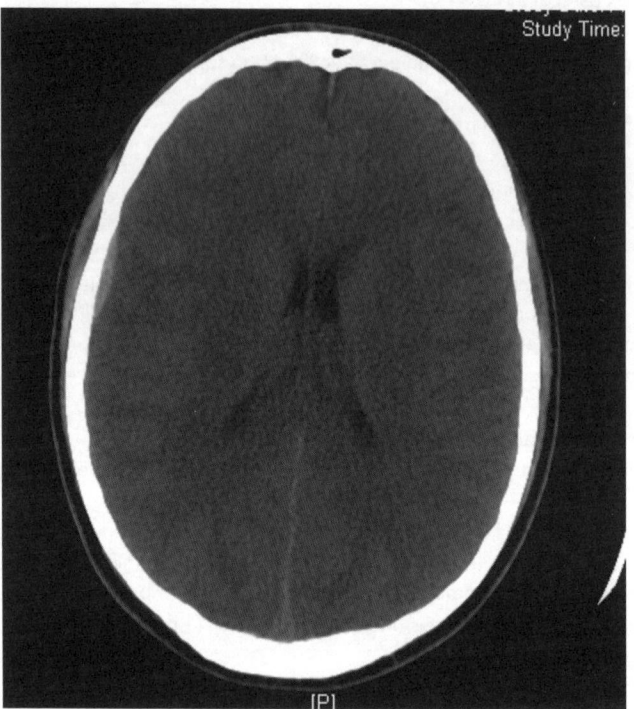

Figure 6.8 CT head

Look at Figure 6.8

a) This CT scan demonstrates a subdural haematoma. (1 mark)

b) This injury can occur in conjunction with a skull fracture. (1 mark)

c) The most commonly injured meningeal vessel is the middle meningeal artery. (1 mark)

d) Subdural haematomas are formed due to tearing of bridging veins between the surface of the brain and the dura. (1 mark)

e) Extradural haematomas occur more commonly than subdural haematomas in patients with a low conscious level. (1 mark)

f) All patients over 65 who suffer a head injury should have a CT. (1 mark)

g) All patients who have vomited following a head injury should have a CT head within 1 hour. (1 mark)

h) The injury in Figure 6.8 is on the right side. (1 mark)

i) 20% Mannitol may be given in a dose of 0.5–1g/kg to reduce intracranial pressure. (1 mark)

j) Prophylactic phenytoin may be used to reduce the incidence of post-traumatic epilepsy. (1 mark)

Answers

Look at Figure 6.8

a) This CT scan demonstrates a subdural haematoma. (1 mark)
- False
  This demonstrates an extradural haematoma.

b) This injury can occur in conjunction with a skull fracture. (1 mark)
- True
  Overlying skull fractures may lacerate meningeal arteries within the epidural space. These can lead to rapidly forming haematomas that may cause rapid deterioration and death. Extradural haematomas are also caused by damage to dural sinuses, which may enlarge more slowly and exert less pressure on the underlying brain.

c) The most commonly injured meningeal vessel is the middle meningeal artery. (1 mark)
- True

d) Subdural haematomas are formed due to tearing of bridging veins between the surface of the brain and the dura. (1 mark)
- True

e) Etradural haematomas occur more commonly than subdural haematomas in patients with a low conscious level. (1 mark)
- False
  Extradural haematomas occur in 9% of patients following head injury who are comatosed, whereas subdural haematomas occur in 30% of severe brain injuries.

f) All patients over 65 who suffer a head injury should have a CT. (1 mark)
- False
  According to National Institute for Health and Clinical Excellence (NICE) guidelines all patients over 65 who have experienced an episode of loss of consciousness or amnesia following a head injury should have a CT scan.

g) All patients who have vomited following a head injury should have a CT head within 1 hour. (1 mark)
- False
  NICE guidelines state that more than 1 episode of vomiting in adults is an indication for a CT head within 1 hour.

h) The injury in Figure 6.8 is on the right side. (1 mark)
- True
  The extradural haematoma is on the right.

i) 20% Mannitol may be given in a dose of 0.5–1g/kg to reduce intracranial pressure. (1 mark)
- True
  Indications for giving mannitol include a dilated, non-responsive pupil, a raised ICP (if monitoring is *in situ*) or a clinical suspicion that the patient is 'coning' i.e. Cushing's reflex. The administration of mannitol should be discussed with the neurosurgical team and decompressive surgery may be required.

j) Prophylactic phenytoin may be used to reduce the incidence of post-traumatic epilepsy. (1 mark)
- False

A loading dose of 1g of phenytoin over 20minutes, followed by 100mg total dissolved solids (TDS) may be used to reduce seizure activity for the first week following injury. Unfortunately, this has not been found to reduce the incidence of long-term epilepsy, which occurs in 15% of all patients who survive following a severe head injury.

Further reading

Hopkins, R Peden, C, Gandhi S. *Radiology for Anaesthesia and Intensive Care* (2nd edn). Cambridge University Press, 2009

Chapter 7 **Equipment**

Introduction

These stations assess your knowledge of certain pieces of equipment and skills to perform basic safety checks on them. This chapter is written with that in mind; asking you to identify key pieces of equipment, with further questioning on safety checks, as well as required knowledge.

In reality you will often be asked to perform checks or assemble circuits but as this work book is designed to be used for independent study these practical skills can be questioned only, therefore it is important to use this book to consolidate knowledge and then practice the required skill.

There will be one equipment station in the OSCE.

1. Filters

Questions

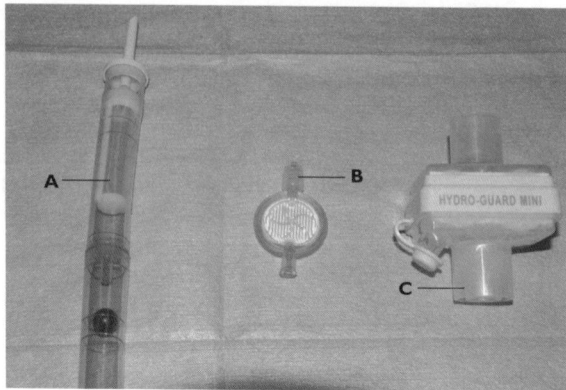

Figure 7.1 Filters. Please see colour plate section.

Look at Figure 7.1

a) What is A? (1 mark)
b) What type of filter is it? (2 marks)
c) What is the purpose of this filter? (2 marks)
d) What is B? (1 mark)
e) What is the purpose of this filter? (2 marks)
f) What type of filter is it? (2 marks)
g) What is the pore size? (2 marks)
h) What is C? (1 mark)
i) Would it be appropriate for a 10kg child? (3 marks)
j) Rank the organisms in Table 7.1 in order of size (biggest =1 to smallest=4). (4 marks)

Table 7.1 Organisms to be ranked in size order

Organism	Rank
Mycobacterium tuberculosis	
Human Immunodeficiency Virus (HIV)	
Staphlococcus aureus	
Hepatitis C virus	

Answers

Look at Figure 7.1

a) What is A? (1 mark)
  • Blood giving set
b) What type of filter is it? (2 marks)
  • Large particle filter
c) What is the purpose of this filter? (2 marks)
  • Prevents large clots and micro aggregates passing to the patient
d) What is B? (1 mark)
  • Epidural filter
e) What is the purpose of this filter? (2 marks)
  • Filtration of bacteria and foreign bodies
f) What type of filter is it? (2 marks)
  • Hydrophilic
g) What is the pore size? (2 marks)
  • 0.22-micron mesh
h) What is C? (1 mark)
  • HME (heat and moisture exchange) filter
i) Would it be appropriate for a 10kg child? (3 marks)
  • No. As an adult HME, it would create too much dead space for a 10kg child
j) Rank the organisms in Table 7.1 in order of size (biggest =1 to smallest=4) (4 marks)
  • Please see complete answer in Table 7.2.

Table 7.2 Organisms to be ranked in size order

Organism	Rank
Mycobacterium tuberculosis	2 (0.3 micron)
HIV	3 (0.08 micron)
Staphlococcus aureus	1 (1 micron)
Hepatitis C virus	4 (0.02 micron)

2. Cylinders

Questions

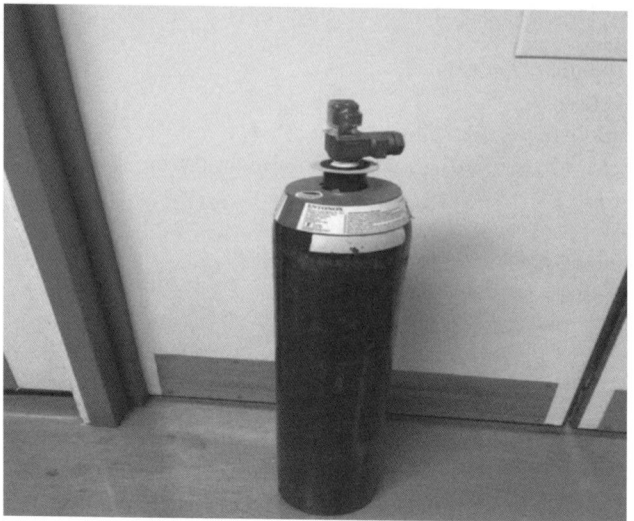

Figure 7.2 Cylinder. Please see colour plate section.

Look at Figure 7.2

a) What is stored in this cylinder? (1 mark)
b) What are the constituents of this? (1 mark)
c) What is attached to this cylinder to allow delivery of gas? (1 mark)
d) What is the pressure within these cylinders? (1 mark)
e) What does the term 'pseudocritical temperature' mean? (2 marks)
f) What is the 'Poynting effect'? (2 marks)
g) Can a hypoxic mixture be delivered? (2 marks)
h) How should cylinders be stored? (1 mark)
i) Name the pin index and colours of the cylinders in Table 7.3. (4 marks)
j) List 4 pieces of information engraved on cylinders. (2 marks)
k) List 3 methods of testing a cylinder. (3 marks)

Table 7.3 Cylinder pin index and colour

Gas	Cylinder colour	PIN index
Oxygen		
Air		
Nitrous Oxide		
Helium		

Answers

Look at Figure 7.2

a) What is stored in this cylinder? (1 mark)
- Entonox

b) What are the constituents of this? (1 mark)
- A compressed gas mixture containing 50% oxygen and 50% nitrous oxide by volume

c) What is attached to this cylinder to allow delivery of gas? (1 mark)
- A two-stage pressure demand regulator. As the patient inspires through the mouth piece gas flow is allowed to occur

d) What is the pressure within these cylinders? (1 mark)
- 13700KPa, or 137 ba

e) What does the term 'pseudocritical temperature' mean? (2 marks)
- This is the temperature at which a mixture of gases separates. For entonox this occurs at −5.5°C, at 117 bar and at -30°C, at 4.1bar

f) What is the 'Poynting effect'? (2 marks)
- The production of a gaseous mixture of oxygen and nitrous oxide by bubbling oxygen through liquid nitrous oxide, causing vaporisation of the liquid

g) Can a hypoxic mixture be delivered? (2 marks)
- Yes. When separation of the gaseous mixture occurs, a high oxygen concentration gas will be delivered initially followed by a gas with an ever-decreasing oxygen concentration as the liquid nitrous oxide evaporates. Rewarming can reverse the separation

h) How should cylinders be stored? (1 mark)
- Horizontally for 24hr at temperatures of 5°C or above before use. Large cylinders have a dip tube to use liquid nitrous oxide therefore preventing a hypoxic mixture

i) Name the pin index and colours of the cylinders in Table 7.4 (4 marks)
- Please see complete answer in Table 7.4

Table 7.4 Cylinder pin index and colour

Gas	Cylinder colour	PIN index
Oxygen	Black body White shoulders	2 + 5
Air	Black body Black and white checked shoulders	1 + 5
Nitrous Oxide	French blue body French blue shoulders	3 + 5
Helium	Brown body Brown shoulders	2 + 4

j) List 4 pieces of information engraved on cylinders. (2 marks)
- Serial number
- Tare weight
- Test pressure
- Date of testing

k) List 3 methods of testing a cylinder. (2 marks)
- Endoscopic examination (for cracks)
- Tensile testing
- Pressure testing (up to 22000KPa)

3. Rotameters

Questions

a) What type of flowmeter is a Rotameter? (2 marks)

b) Does it measure flow directly or indirectly? (1 mark)

c) What are the components of a Rotameter? (4 marks)

d) What theory about gas flow allows measurement of flow with a Rotameter? (3 marks)

e) Describe how flow is different at low and high flow rates. (5 marks)

f) Why do you need different Rotameters for different gases? (1 mark)

g) Where do you read the bobbin and the ball on a Rotatmeter? (1 mark)

h) How does the Rotameter overcome friction? (2 marks)

i) How would an increase in temperature affect measurement of the flow at low flow rates in a Rotameter? (1 mark)

Answers

a) What type of flowmeter is a Rotameter? (2 marks)
   - It is a constant pressure, variable orifice device
b) Does it measure flow directly or indirectly? (1 mark)
   - It is an indirect measure
c) What are the components of a Rotameter? (4 marks)
   - a vertical tapered tube, wider at the top than the bottom
   - a floating bobbin or ball
   - a valve at the bottom which controls flow into the tube
   - a scale representing flow rate
d) What theory about gas flow allows measurement of flow with a Rotameter? (3 marks)
   - There is a constant pressure across the bobbin at all levels of the tube but there is variable resistance to flow depending on the diameter of the tube
e) Describe how flow is different at low and high flow rates (5 marks)
   - At low flow rates, flow is laminar (tube effect). Therefore, flow can be described by the Hagen-Poiseuille equation and is viscosity dependent

$$Q= (P\pi r4) /(8\eta l)$$

   Q= flow, P=pressure, r=radius, η=viscosity, l=length
   - At high flow rates, flow is turbulent because of the wider diameter of the tube (orifice effect). The variable nature of turbulent flow means that there is no exact formula, but flow is dependent on the density of the gas and the square root of the pressure drop
f) Why do you need different Rotameters for different gases? (1 mark)
   - Different gases have different density and viscosities therefore the flow past the bobbin is gas dependent
g) Where do you read the bobbin and the ball on a Rotatmeter? (1 mark)
   - A bobbin is read from the top and the ball from the widest diameter
h) How does the Rotameter overcome friction? (2 marks)
   - The bobbin is skirted so that it spins when gas flows past preventing it from 'sticking' to the side of the tube
   - The tubes are coated with tin oxide to allow electrostatic forces to be earthed
i) How would an increase in temperature affect measurement of the flow at low flow rates in a Rotameter? (1 mark)
   - An increase in temperature leads to an increase in viscosity but a decrease in density, therefore at lower flows there would be an over reading

4. Bain circuit

Questions

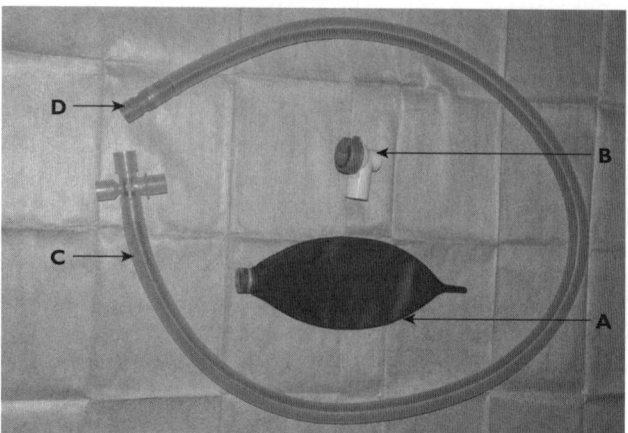

Figure 7.3 Circuit components. Please see colour plate section.

Look at Figure 7.3

a) Of which circuit are these the component parts? (1 mark)

b) Assemble circuit by filling in the blanks. (4 marks)

$$\text{FGF} \rightarrow \quad \begin{array}{c} \uparrow \\ \\ \downarrow \end{array} \quad \longrightarrow \quad \longrightarrow \text{patient}$$

c) How would you examine the circuit to ensure it was safe to use? (8 marks)

d) What is the minimum gas flow required during the following?
   i) Controlled ventilation (1 mark)
   ii) Spontaneous ventilation (1 mark)

e) What effect would a hole in the reservoir bag have in spontaneous ventilation? (1 mark)

f) What is the effect of the internal tubing becoming disconnected? (1 mark)

g) What is the effect of an increase in tubing length? (1 mark)

h) Where and how can a ventilator be attached to this circuit? (2 marks)

Answers

Look at Figure 7.3

a) Of which circuit are these the component parts? (1 mark)
- Bain circuit

b) Assemble circuit by filling in the blanks. (4 marks)

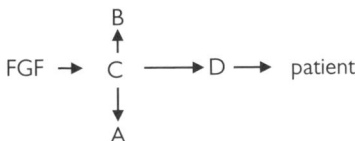

c) How would you examine the circuit to ensure it was safe to use? (8 marks)
- Visual inspection. Ensure assembled correctly, no tears in the reservoir bag, no crack in the outer tubing and that the inner tubing has not become disconnected
- Inner tubing. Turn oxygen flow up and occlude the inner tube with the plunger from a 2ml syringe. Integrity is confirmed by the bobbin dropping due to back pressure
- Outer tubing. Occlude the outer tubing with your thumb filling reservoir bag then squeeze the bag feeling the increase in pressure or turn the gas flow down and ensure that the bag does not collapse
- Pethicks test. Close adjustable pressure limiting (APL) valve and fill bag and breathing system using the oxygen flush whilst occluding the outer tubing with your thumb. Then release occlusion whilst still pressing the oxygen flush and the venturi effect will cause the bag to collapse.

d) What is the minimum gas flow required during the following?
  i) Controlled ventilation (1 mark)
  - 1 x minute ventilation (approximately 5Litres/min)
  ii) Spontaneous ventilation (1 mark)
  - 2–3 x minute ventilation (approximately 15Litres/min in a 70Kg patient)

e) What effect would a hole in the reservoir bag have in spontaneous ventilation? (1 mark)
- No effect as long as the fresh gas flow remains greater than minute ventilation. You may also lose the movement of the bag as a visual representation of spontaneous ventilation

f) What is the effect of the internal tubing becoming disconnected? (1 mark)
- Increased dead space which can lead to hypoxaemia and hypercapnoea

g) What is the effect of an increase in tubing length? (1 mark)
- Does not affect properties but can cause some increase in resistance to expiration in spontaneous ventilation

h) Where and how can a ventilator be attached to this circuit? (2 marks)
- Remove the reservoir bag and close the APL valve. Attach 1 metre of corrugated tubing (volume of tubing must be more than 500ml to prevent driving pressure from the ventilator being applied to the patient)

5. Laryngoscopes and tubes

Questions

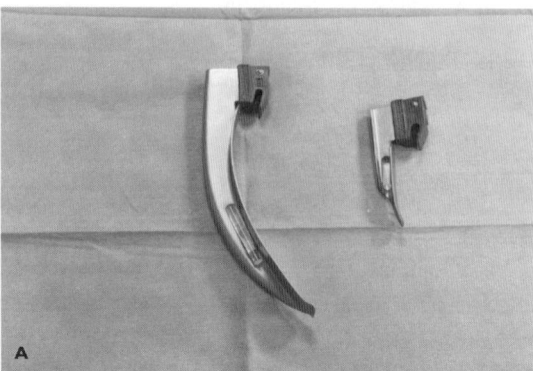

Figure 7.4a Laryngoscopes. Please see colour plate section.

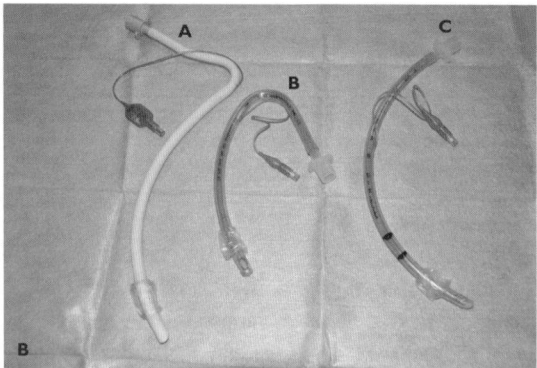

Figure 7.4b Tubes. Please see colour plate section.

a) Look at Figures 7.4a and b. Name the items. (1 marks)
b) Identify 4 physical differences between them. (4 marks)
c) Describe the haemodynamic response to intubation. (2 marks)
d) Which nerve mediates the bradycardic response to intubation in children? (1 mark)
e) Describe 2 differences between fibre optic laryngoscopes and conventional blades with a bulb. (2 marks)
f) What precautions would you need to take when using a laryngoscope in the MRI scanner? (1 mark)
Look at Figure 7.4b
g) What are A, B and C? (1 mark)
h) List 2 practical measures to reduce the risk of trauma when inserting A. (2 marks)
i) What is the formula to calculate the correct internal diameter (ID) tube size? (2 marks)
j) What is the formula to calculate the correct length of the tube? (2 marks)
k) List an advantage and disadvantage of using B over C. (2 marks)

Answers

a) Look at Figures 7.4a and b. Name the items. (2 marks)
- A = Adult Macintosh laryngoscope
- B = Paediatric Miller laryngoscope

b) Identify 4 physical differences between them. (4 marks)
- Curved blade on Macintosh versus straight blade of Miller
- Size 3 adult MAC blade and size 1 infant Miller blade
- The tip of the MAC blade is designed to fit into the vallecula and is therefore bulbous to help lift the larynx whilst the straight blade has a slight upturned tip and is designed to pass over the posterior border of the epiglottis to give a view of the larynx
- MAC flange is a large reverse Z shape whilst Miller flange is a compressed short D shape

c) Describe the haemodynamic response to intubation? (2 marks)
- Increase in heart rate and blood pressure (both systolic and diastolic)

d) Which nerve mediates the bradycardic response to intubation in children? (1 mark)
- Vagus nerve

e) Describe 2 differences between fibre optic laryngoscopes and conventional blades with a bulb? (2 marks)
- Conventional laryngoscopes have the bulb on the blade and fibre optic (or more accurately – fibre lit, as fibre optic bundles are often not used) have the light source on the handle
- In conventional laryngoscopes the light comes on when an electrical connection is made between the blade and the handle (making it quite robust but it could flicker and may need changing). In fibre optic laryngoscopes there is a light conducting fibre (glass or plastic) which converges light from the top of the handle to the distal portion of the blade

f) What precautions would you need to take when using a laryngoscope in the MRI scanner? (1 mark)
- Ensure it is plastic and not made of ferrous metal

Look at Figure 7.5b

g) What are A, B and C? (1 mark)
- A – Nasal endotracheal tube
- B – South facing Ring, Adair, Elwyn (RAE) endotracheal tube
- C – Endotracheal tube

h) List 2 practical measures to reduce the risk of trauma when inserting A. (2 marks)
- Apply local anaesthetic to the nasal passage and use a series of dilators to dilate the nasopharynx before insertion of the nasal exercise tolerance testing (ETT). Warm the tip of the nasal tube to soften it before insertion. Once the tube has passed into the oropharynx, use a laryngoscope and Magill's forceps to guide the tube through the larynx
- Pass the nasal tube through a nasopharyngeal airway preventing the hard tip of the tube from causing trauma in the nasopharynx. The nasopharyngeal airway can be removed once the tube has been placed

i) What is the formula to calculate the correct internal diameter (ID) tube size? (2 marks)
- $\dfrac{age}{4} + 4$ (uncuffed tube) or $\dfrac{age}{4} + 3.5$ (cuffed tube)

j) What is the formula to calculate the correct length of the tube? (2 marks)
- $\dfrac{age}{2} + 12$ or 3 x tube size (ID) [age / 2 + 15 for nasal tubes]

k) List an advantage and disadvantage using of B over C. (2 marks)
- Advantage: B offers good surgical access to the oropharynx in ENT surgery
- Disadvantage: as B is preformed there is an increased risk of bronchial intubation. As a result, the uncuffed version has two murphy's eyes as this risk is greatest in small children. Conversely a preformed tube may be too short in tall adults

6. Epidurals

Questions

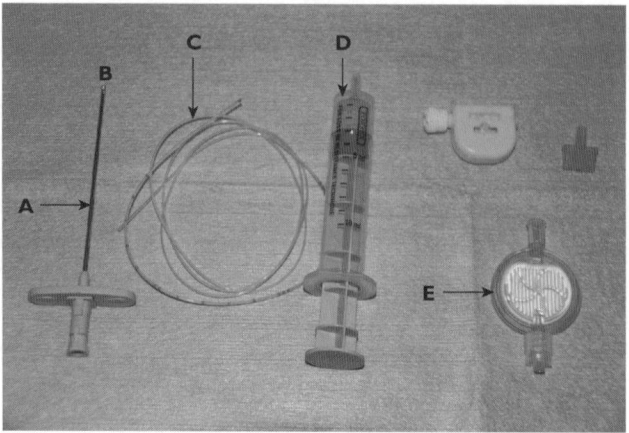

Figure 7.5 Epidurals. Please see colour plate section.

Look at Figure 7.5

a) What is A? (1 mark)

b) What is B? (1 mark)

c) How and why is B shaped as it is? (2 marks)

d) What are the markings on the shaft of the needle called? (1 mark)

e) What is the normal length of the needle and how far apart are the markings? (2 marks)

f) What is C? List 3 of its characteristics. (2 marks)

g) What is special about D? (1 mark)

h) What volume is required to prime E? (1 mark)

i) What will A pass through before reaching the epidural space? (5 marks)

j) When using a lumbar epidural, what volume of local anaesthetic is required for a block to prime? (2 marks)

k) Why do labouring women require less local anaesthetic to achieve the same block? (2 marks)

Answers

Look at Figure 7.5

a) What is A? (1 mark)
- Tuohy needle

b) What is B? (1 mark)
- Huber tip

c) How and why is B shaped as it is? (2 marks)
- How: blunt and oblique (20 degrees to the shaft)
- Why: To reduce the risk of dural puncture and to allow the catheter to be directed by the operator (caudal or cephalic)

d) What are the markings on the shaft of the needle called? (1 mark)
- Lee's lines

e) What is the normal length of the needle and how far apart are the markings? (2 marks)
- Length: 10cm with shaft of 8cm (5 and 15cm needles also exist)
- Distance between markings: 1cm

f) What is C? List 3 of its characteristics. (2 marks)
- C = Epidural catheter
- It is a 90cm flexible, transparent, biologically inert catheter
- Rounded distal tip (reducing the risk of dural or vascular puncture)
- 5cm markings on catheter with 1cm markings between 5 and 15cm
- 2–3 side ports towards distal end but not at tip

g) What is special about D? (1 mark)
- It is a loss of resistance syringe. It has a low resistance plunger allowing identification of the epidural space by loss of resistance to saline (or less commonly air)

h) What volume is required to prime E? (1 mark)
- This is a hydrophilic filter with 0.22micron mesh and requires a minimum volume of 0.7ml to prime

i) What will A pass through before reaching the epidural space? (5 marks)
- Skin
- Subcutaneous tissue
- Supraspinous ligament
- Interspinous ligament
- Ligamentum flavum

j) When using a lumbar epidural, what volume of local anaesthetic is required for a block to prime? (2 marks)
- T10 = 10–12ml
- T4 = 20–25ml

k) Why do labouring women require less local anaesthetic to achieve the same block? (2 marks)
- Venous distension reduces the volume of the epidural space
- An increase in circulating progesterone increases nerve sensitivity to local anaesthetic

7. Scavenging

Questions

a) What two functions does a scavenging system provide? (2 marks)

b) Name 2 types of scavenging system. (2 marks)

c) Describe the difference between them. (2 marks)

d) List the 4 main components of a scavenging system. (4 marks)

e) What size connector is attached to the tubing which transports the gases to the scavenging system (transfer tubing)? (1 mark)

f) How and what values are positive and negative pressure limited to within a scavenging system? (3 marks)

g) Name 6 ways to reduce pollution in theatre. (3 marks)

h) How many air changes should occur in a theatre environment? (1 mark)

i) What are the maximum accepted concentrations in the UK over an 8 hour period for nitrous oxide and isoflurane? (2 marks)

Answers

a) What two functions does a scavenging system provide? (2 marks)
- Collects waste anaesthetic gas
- Disposes of waste gas safely

b) Name 2 types of scavenging system. (2 marks)
- Active scavenging
- Passive scavenging

c) Describe the difference between them. (2 marks)
- In an active system the exhaled gases are driven by a vacuum (produced either by a pump or by a motorised fan); the ventilator or the patient's respiration drives a passive system
- As such the active system is able to cope with a wider range of expiratory flow rates and there is less risk of reverse flow that can occur in a passive system

d) List the 4 main components of a scavenging system. (4 marks)
- Collecting system
- Transfer system
- Receiving system
- Disposal system

e) What size connector is attached to the tubing which transports the gases to the scavenging system (transfer tubing)? (1 mark)
- 30mm. This is to prevent misconnections with breathing circuits. The transfer tubing is also 30mm

f) How and what values are positive and negative pressure limited to within a scavenging system? (3 marks)
- How is pressure limited? Loaded valves protect against excessive pressure
- Positive pressure limit = 1000 Pa
- Negative pressure limit = −50 Pa

g) Name 6 ways to reduce pollution in theatre. (3 marks)
- Adequate theatre ventilation
- Use of circle breathing system
- Scavenging
- Total Intravenous anaesthesia
- Regional anaesthesia
- Cautious filling of vaporisers to prevent spillage

h) How many air changes should occur in a theatre environment? (1 mark)
- Traditionally in the UK 15–20 air changes per hour

  2007 DOH guidelines suggest up to 25 changes per hour with a minimum of 18. The supply air should be filtered to EN779 F7 standard and there should be a positive pressure differential of 25 Pa compared with outside air.

i) What are the maximum accepted concentrations in the UK over an 8 hour period for nitrous oxide and isoflurane? (2 marks)
- Nitrous oxide 100 particles per million
- Isoflurane 50 particles per million

  Control of substances hazardous to health (COSHH) 2002 over an 8 hour time period)

8. Suction

Questions

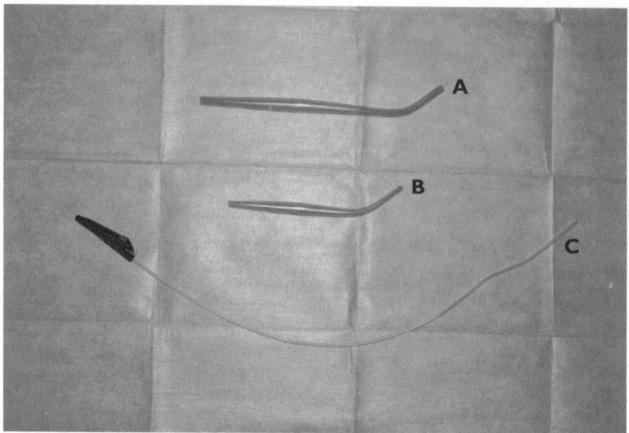

Figure 7.6 Suction. Please see colour plate section.

a) List 5 uses for suction in anaesthesia. (5 marks)
b) Define the terms 'suction' and 'vacuum'. (2 marks)
c) What three parts comprise a centralised vacuum system? (3 marks)
d) List three requirements that should be met by each anaesthetic room suction outlet. (3 marks)
Look at Figure 7.6
e) Name the following. (3 marks)
f) Name 4 hazards posed by suction systems. (4 marks)

Answers

a) List 5 uses for suction in anaesthesia. (5 marks)
- Clearing the airway (trachea, oropharynx, bronchoscopy)
- Pleural suction (-3kPa) and other systems connected to drains
- Gastric decompression/emptying
- Cardio-pulmonary bypass
- Gas scavenging

b) Define the terms 'suction' and 'vacuum'. (2 marks)
- Suction: The application of negative pressure to move gases, liquids and/or solids
- Vacuum: a space entirely devoid of matter

c) What three parts comprise a centralised vacuum system? (3 marks)
- Pump
- Receiver
- Filter

d) List three requirements that should be met by each anaesthetic room suction outlet. (3 marks)
- A maximum negative pressure of -52kPa (some sources say -60kPa) or -400mmHg
- 40L/min free air flow
- 4 second time constant (i.e. reaches 65% of final within 4 seconds)

e) Name the following. (3 marks)
- A – Adult Yankauer sucker
- B – Paediatric Yankauer sucker
- C – Suction catheter

f) Name 4 hazards posed by suction systems. (4 marks)
- Kinking/obstruction of catheter
- Trauma (to trachea/oropharynx) from catheters/Yankauers
- Disconnection, unavailability when required
- Excessive suction (e.g. chest drains)
- Health hazard to those cleaning equipment used for suctioning

9. Depth of anaesthesia

Questions

a) Fill in the missing words in this explanation of the 'isolated forearm technique'. (6 marks)

A patient is anaesthetised.

A .... is placed on the patient's ....…............... and inflated above ....

....

A .... is then administered.

The patient's depth of anaesthesia can be assessed ....…….... by the anaesthetist.

If the patient is aware, or in pain, they are able to squeeze ....

b) Name 3 disadvantages of the isolated forearm technique. (3 marks)

c) How does BIS monitoring technique work? (3 marks)

d) What do the numbers 0 and 100, related to this technique, represent respectively? (2 marks)

e) What range is considered to represent surgical/general anaesthesia when using this technique? (1 mark)

f) What is the significance of burst suppression? (1 mark)

g) Name 4 other methods of depth of anaesthesia monitoring? (4 marks)

Answers

a) Fill in the missing words in this explanation of the 'isolated forearm technique'. (6 marks)

A patient is anaesthetised.
A *pneumatic cuff/tourniquet* is placed on the patient's *upper arm* and inflated above *systolic pressure*.
A *neuromuscular blocking agent* is then administered.
The patient's depth of anaesthesia can be assessed *using direct questioning* by the anaesthetist.
If the patient is aware, or in pain, they are able to squeeze *the anaesthetist's hand*.

b) Name 3 disadvantages of the isolated forearm technique. (3 marks)
- Patient cooperation needed
- Spontaneous movement of the arm interferes with interpretation of this technique
- Duration of cuff inflation must be limited for two reasons:
  - Patient discomfort, skin changes, pressure sores
  - After 20mins, ischaemic paralysis of the forearm may occur, preventing movement

c) How does BIS monitoring technique work? (3 marks)
- Analysis and comparison of modified electroencephalogram (EEG) frequencies to produce a scale representing the transition between consciousness and unconsciousness
- Monitored by the anaesthetist during anaesthesia and used as a guide to titrate anaesthetic

d) What do the following numbers, related to this technique, represent respectively? (2 marks)
- 0: Cortical electrical silence
- 100: normal cortical activity (awake patient)

e) What range is considered to represent surgical/general anaesthesia when using this technique? (1 mark)
- 40–60

f) What is the significance of burst suppression? (1 mark)
- Frequent burst suppression suggests the patient is too heavily or 'over' anaesthetised

g) Name 4 other methods of depth of anaesthesia monitoring. (4 marks)
- Clinical signs (e.g. heart rate, blood pressure, respiratory rate, sweating, pupils)
- Respiratory and skeletal muscle activity (e.g. frequency and depth of respiration, skeletal muscle response to surgical stimulation)
- Degree of sympathetic stimulation (physical review special topics [PRST scoring system). Score allocated to four variables and the total used to indicate degree of sympathetic stimulation and therefore depth of anaesthesia. Variables are: systolic arterial Pressure, Pulse rate, Sweating, Tear formation. Not shown to provide any benefit in detecting awareness
- Evoked potentials (visual, somatosensory, auditory – last to disappear)
- EEG interpretation (limited value, complex)
- Respiratory sinus arrhythmia (note need intact autonomic nervous system and healthy myocardial conducting system)
- Oesophageal contractility – amplitude and frequency of contractions of lower oesophageal smooth muscle reduce with increasing depth of anaesthesia. High rate of false positive and false negative results. Affected by relaxants and oesophageal disease
- Frontalis (scalp) electrocardiogram (EMG) – Amplitude of EMG measured. Decreases with increasing depth of anaesthesia. Not useful in paralysed patients

10. Pacemakers

Questions

Look at Figure 7.7a

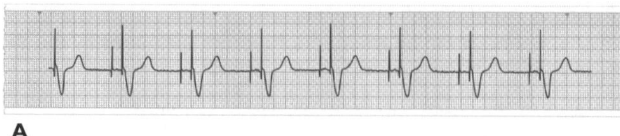

A

Figure 7.7a ECG. Please see colour plate section.

ECG, Courtesy of Dr Oliver Meyer

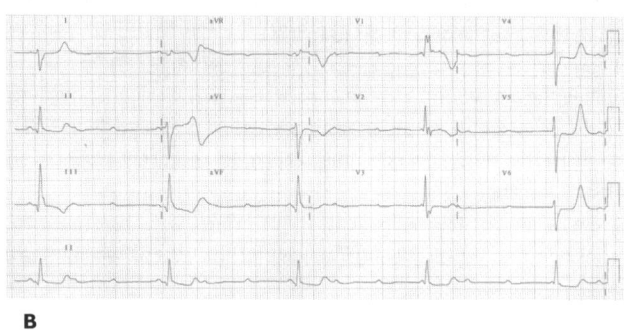

B

Figure 7.7b ECG. Please see colour plate section.

Reproduced from Myerson SG et al., *Emergencies in Cardiology*, 2009 with permission from Oxford University Press

a) What do the ECGs show? Explain the ECG features to support your answer. (4 marks)
Look at Figure 7.7b

b) How could you treat a patient whose ECG looked like Figure 7.7b? (2 marks)

Look at Figure 7.7c

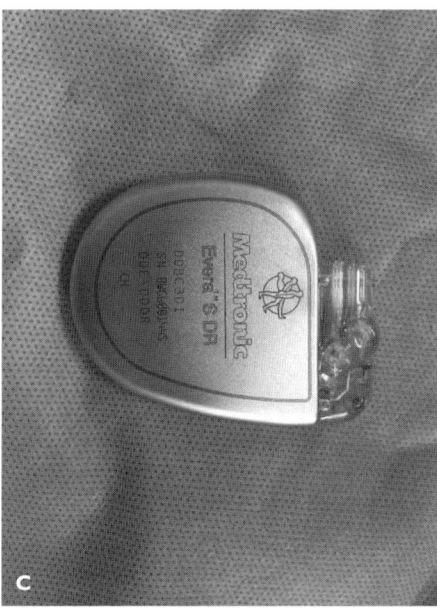

Figure 7.7c Defibrillator. Please see colour plate section

c) What is it? (1 mark)

d) What is its function? (1 mark)

e) Considering pacing, how and where anatomically is a temporary pacing wire inserted? (2 marks)

f) Name three indications for pacemaker insertion. (3 marks)

g) With respect to pacemaker generic codes, explain what function a VVI pacemaker will perform? (4 marks)

h) Name three pieces of equipment in a hospital setting that may interfere with pacemaker function. (3 marks)

Answers

Look at Figure 7.7a.

a) What do the ECGs show? Explain the ECG features to support your answer. (4 marks)
- Figure 7.7a: ECG showing paced rhythm. Pacing spikes, wide QRS complexes
- Figure 7.7b: ECG showing third-degree (complete) AV block. P waves and QRS complexes are independent of each other

Look at Figure 7.7b

b) How could you treat a patient whose ECG looked like Figure 7.7b? (2 marks)
- Cardiac pacing
- Could be achieved: externally, transcutaneously or transvenously

Look at Figure 7.7c

c) What is it? (1 mark)
- Internal Cardiac Defibrillator

d) What is its function? (1 mark)
- To detect and terminate abnormal rhythms

e) Considering pacing, how and where anatomically is a temporary pacing wire inserted? (2 marks)
- Through the subclavian, jugular or femoral vein into the right ventricle
- X-ray screening is required to guide placement
- Must take place with full resuscitation equipment immediately available

f) Name three indications for pacemaker insertion. (3 marks)
- Sinus node problems e.g. sick sinus syndrome, recurrent Stoke-Adams syndrome, sinus node dysfunction
- Chronic arrhythmias e.g. atrial fibrillation
- Complete AV block (third-degree heart block)
- Symptomatic second degree AV block
- Atrio-biventricular pacing in moderate to severe heart failure

g) With respect to pacemaker generic codes, explain what function a VVI pacemaker will perform? (4 marks)
- First letter indicates the chamber paced: atrium (A), ventricle (V), dual (D), none (O)
- Second letter indicates the chamber sensed: atrium (A), ventricle (V), dual (D), none (O)
- Third letter indicates response to sensing: triggered (T), inhibited (I), dual (D, none (O))
- Fourth letter indicates rate modulation or programmability: rate modulated (R), communicating (C), multi programmable (M), simple programmable (P), none (O)
- Fifth letter describes anti-tachycardia function: paced (P), shocks (S), dual (D)
- So a VVI pacemaker will pace the ventricle, sense the ventricle and respond by inhibiting it (i.e. if the ventricle stops contracting the pacemaker will pace at a set rhythm, stopping only when it senses a spontaneous ventricular contraction.)

h) Name three pieces of equipment in a hospital setting that may interfere with pacemaker function. (3 marks)
- Diathermy (especially monopolar)
- Nerve stimulators
- MRI
- Central venous catheters, pulmonary artery catheters – physical dislodgement of wires

Further reading

Al-Shaikh B, Stacey S. *Essentials of Anaesthetic Equipment* (3rd edn). Churchill Livingstone, 2–4, 10–11, 41–2, 52–6, 125–7, 184–6, 2008

Davis P, Kenny G. *Basic Physics and Measurement in Anaesthesia* (5th edn). Butterworth Heinmann, 49, 249–52, 2007

Deakin C. *Clinical Notes for the FRCA*. Churchill Livingstone, 348–53, 2011

Chapter 8 **Hazards**

Introduction

The 'Hazards' question tests the way in which harm may be caused to patients of staff in the operating theatre. There may be significant overlap with the 'Hazards' question and the physics section of the Structured Oral Examination.

1. Blood transfusion

Questions

a) What should be documented in the notes before transfusing blood? (3 marks)

b) Write down the checks you would complete before transfusing blood into a patient? (8 marks)

c) What are you looking for when you inspect a blood bag? (3 marks)

d) During what time frame does a transfusion of red cells need to be started following removal from the fridge? (1 mark)

e) During what time frame does the transfusion of red cells need to be completed following removal from the fridge? (1 mark)

f) What is the most common complication of blood transfusion? (1 mark)

g) What are the clinical features of a reaction to a blood product while under anaesthesia? (3 marks)

Answers

a) What should be documented in the notes before transfusing blood? (3 marks)
   - Reason for transfusion
   - Blood component to be given
   - Patient has been informed of the intended transfusion

b) Write down the checks you would complete before transfusing blood into a patient? (8 marks)
   - Check for a valid prescription
   - Ensure special requirements are met, for example cytomegalovirus (CMV) negative
   - Inspect the bag
   - Patient states full name and date of birth and these match their wrist ID band
   - Check the ID band matches the compatibility label on the blood product
   - Check the details on the compatibility label match the blood product and check that the compatibility label matches the form that comes with the blood (if present)
   - Sign, date and time the form

c) What are you looking for when you inspect a blood bag? (3 marks)

   Any 3 of:
   - Expiry date
   - Discolouration
   - Clumping
   - Leaks

d) During what time frame does a transfusion of red cells need to be started following removal from the fridge? (1 mark)
   - Within 30 minutes

e) During what time frame does the transfusion of red cells need to be completed following removal from the fridge? (1 mark)
   - 4 hours

f) What is the most common complication of blood transfusion? (1 mark)
   - Non-haemolytic febrile reaction

g) What are the clinical features of a reaction to a blood product while under anaesthesia? (3 marks)

   Any 3 of:
   - Hypotension
   - Tachycardia
   - Hyperthermia
   - Tachypnoea if breathing spontaneously
   - Urticaria

2. Defibrillation

Questions

a) State 3 indications for defibrillation. (3 marks)

b) What is the advantage of biphasic defibrillation? (1 mark)

c) Summarise the energy transferred in terms of voltage and charge. (1 mark)

d) State Ohm's law and write an equation representing this. (2 marks)

e) What is impedance? (2 marks)

f) Name 2 factors that may affect impedance when using a defibrillator (2 marks)

g) What is capacitance? (1 mark)

h) Draw a simple discharging defibrillator circuit incorporating a power source, switches, a capacitor and a patient. (3 marks)

i) What is the purpose of the inductor within the circuit? (1 mark)

j) State 3 steps that can be taken to ensure safety when delivering a shock. (3 marks)

Answers

a) State 3 indications for defibrillation. (3 marks)

Any 3 of:
- Supraventricular tachycardia with cardiac compromise
- Ventricular tachycardia with cardiac compromise
- Pulseless ventricular tachycardia
- Ventricular fibrillation

b) What is the advantage of biphasic defibrillation? (1 mark)
- Reduction in the energy required thus reducing the risk of burns and myocardial damage

c) Summarise the energy transferred in terms of voltage and charge. (1 mark)
- E=QV (Energy= charge x voltage)

d) State Ohm's law and write an equation representing this. (2 marks)
- The current flowing through a conductor between 2 points is directly proportional to the potential difference and inversely proportional to the resistance
- V=IR or I=V/R

e) What is impedance? (2 marks)
- Impedance is a measure of the total opposition to alternating current flow
- It consists of both resistance and reactance

f) Name 2 factors that may affect impedance when using a defibrillator. (2 marks)

Any 2 of:
- Increased body mass
- Phase of ventilation – lowest on full expiration
- Presence of lung disease e.g. emphysema
- Interface between the electrodes and the skin
- Electrode size
- Distance between the electrodes on the chest
- Time elapsed since previous shock

g) What is capacitance? (1 mark)
- The ability of a body to store charge

h) Draw a simple discharging defibrillator circuit incorporating a power source, switches, a capacitor and a patient. (3 marks)

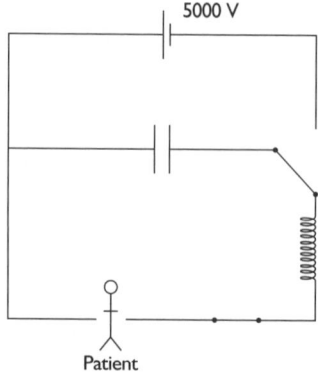

5000 V

Patient

Figure 8.1 Discharging defibrillator circuit

i) What is the purpose of the inductor within the circuit? (2 marks)
- Extends discharge time and ensures a smoother profile (which would otherwise be exponential decay)

j) State 3 steps that can be taken to ensure safety when delivering a shock. (3 marks)

Any 3 of:
- Use of an automated external defibrillator via non-touch electrodes
- Ensure no-one is in contact with the patient via visual sweep of bedside area and verbal command
- Ensure no-one is in contact with any conductor e.g. fluids/ metal
- Remove oxygen sources from the immediate vicinity of the patient

3. Diathermy

Questions

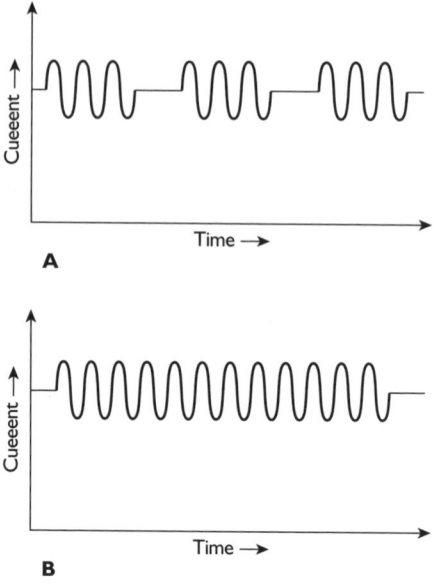

Figure 8.2 Diathermy

Reproduced from Cross ME and Plunket EVE, *Physics, Pharmacology and Physiology for Anaesthetists: Key concepts for the FRCA,* copyright (2014) with permission from Cambridge University Press

a) Why is an adult diathermy plate larger than a paediatric diathermy plate? (2 marks)
b) Which areas should you avoid when applying the diathermy plate to the patient? (4 marks)
c) How does monopolar diathermy work? (3 marks)
d) How does bipolar diathermy work? (3 marks)
e) Which waveform in Figure 8.2 is used for cutting diathermy and which for coagulation? (1 mark)
f) What frequency range is used for diathermy? (2 marks)
g) Why is this frequency used? (2 marks)
h) In addition to those associated with implantable devices, what hazards may be encountered when using diathermy? (3 marks)

Answers

a) Why is an adult diathermy plate larger than a paediatric diathermy plate? (2 marks)
- The adult plate has a higher surface area, therefore current density that flows is lower
- Risk of burns occurring is less with a lower current density

b) Which areas should you avoid when applying the diathermy plate to the patient? (4 marks)

Any 4 of:
- Bony prominences
- Implanted metal prostheses
- Areas distal to tourniquets
- Pressure points
- Hairy areas
- Scar tissue

c) How does monopolar diathermy work? (3 marks)
- Current flows from the diathermy tip, through the patient to the diathermy pad. The current density is very high close to the diathermy tip, resulting in heating and destruction of the tissues. The current density at the diathermy pad is much lower, and therefore not high enough to produce heating of the tissues and burns

d) How does bipolar diathermy work? (3 marks)
- Current flows from one side of the diathermy forceps to the other, resulting in intense heating and destruction of the tissues in between. There is no need for a diathermy plate

e) Which waveform in figure 8.2 is used for cutting diathermy and which for coagulation? (1 mark)
- A – coagulation, B – cutting

f) What frequency range is used for diathermy? (2 marks)
- High frequency current
- From 500,000Hz to over 1MHz

g) Why is this frequency used? (2 marks)
- It is safer. The threshold for inducing ventricular fibrillation at this frequency is much higher

h) In addition to those associated with implantable devices, what hazards may be encountered when using diathermy? (3 marks)
- Burns – through inadvertent activation of diathermy at an inappropriate time, flow to earth through any metal conductor that the patient is touching, incorrect attachment of a diathermy plate or incorrect plate (paediatric plate on an adult patient)
- Ignition of flammable substances (for example bowel gas)
- Interference with monitoring, for example ECG, transoesophageal Doppler

4. Electrical safety

Questions

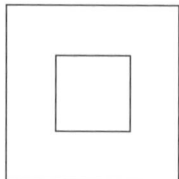

Figure 8.3 Symbol

a) What are the effects of the following currents flowing between the hands at 50Hz (i) 1 mA (ii) 15mA (iii) 75mA? (3 marks)

b) What is microshock? (2 marks)

c) What size current is necessary to induce ventricular fibrillation when applied directly to the myocardium? (1 mark)

d) Give 2 examples of equipment that may produce microshock. (2 marks)

e) State 3 measures to reduce the risk of electrocution in the operating theatre. (3 marks)

f) The classification of electrical equipment refers to the means of protection against electrocution. By what means does class II equipment provide protection? (2 marks)

g) What does the symbol in Figure 8.3 represent? (2 marks)

h) What is Type CF equipment? (2 marks)

i) What is an isolated floating circuit? (3 marks)

Answers

a) What are the effects of the following currents flowing between the hands at 50Hz (i) 1 mA (ii) 15mA (iii) 75mA? (3 marks)
- (i) tingling sensation
- (ii) muscle tetany, pain, asphyxia
- (iii) ventricular fibrillation

b) What is microshock? (2 marks)
- A small current which, when applied directly to the myocardium, has a high current density and can induce ventricular fibrillation

c) What size current is necessary to induce ventricular fibrillation when applied directly to the myocardium? (1 mark)
- 150 MICROamps

d) Give 2 examples of equipment that may produce microshock. (2 marks)

Any 2 of:
- Central venous catheter
- Oesophageal thermometer
- Pacemaker

e) State 3 measures to reduce the risk of electrocution in the operating theatre. (3 marks)
- Ensuring all equipment in the patient environment complies with British Standards for safety
- Regular maintenance and testing of electrical equipment
- Ensuring the patient is not in contact with earthed objects
- Antistatic shoes

f) The classification of electrical equipment refers to the means of protection against electrocution. By what means does class II equipment provide protection? (2 marks)
- Any accessible conducting parts are protected from the live supply by double or reinforced insulation

g) What does this symbol in Figure 8.3 represent? (2 marks)
- Class II equipment

h) What is Type CF equipment? (2 marks)
- Provides the most complete protection, and is suitable for direct cardiac connection
- Utilises a floating circuit and has a maximum leakage current of <10microAmps

i) What is an isolated floating circuit? (3 marks)
- The circuit is connected to the mains via an isolated transformer, that consists of a coil in the mains circuit, and is electrically insulated from a coil in the patient circuit
- When a current is produced in the coil in the mains circuit, it creates an electromagnetic field in the coil in the patient circuit and induces a current
- The mains circuit is earthed, but the patient circuit is not

5. Hand washing

Questions

a) What are the 5 moments of hand-hygiene? (5 marks)

b) According to guidelines, what are the steps involved in hand washing? (8 marks)

c) When is alcohol gel not sufficient for cleaning your hands? (2 marks)

d) Give an example of an organism where you must wash your hands rather than using alcohol hand gel. (1 mark)

e) When should gloves be worn? (4 marks)

Answers

a) What are the 5 moments of hand-hygiene? (5 marks)
- Before patient contact
- Before an aseptic task
- After exposure to body fluids
- After patient contact
- After contact with the patient's surroundings

b) According to guidelines, what are the steps involved in hand washing? (8 marks)
- Wet hands and wrists and apply soap
- Rub palm to palm
- Rub palm to palm with fingers interlaced
- Palm to back of hand with fingers interlaced
- Fingers clasped together
- Rotational rubbing of both thumbs
- Tips of fingers in opposite palm
- Rinse hands with water and dry thoroughly with towel

c) When is alcohol gel not sufficient for cleaning your hands? (2 marks)
- When your hands are visibly soiled
- When there are spore forming organisms present

d) Give an example of an organism where you must wash your hands rather than using alcohol hand gel. (1 mark)
- Clostridium difficile

e) When should gloves be worn? (4 marks)
- Invasive procedures
- Contact with sterile sites, non-intact skin, mucous membranes
- When handling sharps
- Carrying out procedures where there is a risk of exposure to blood or body fluids

6. Lasers

Questions

a) What features of a laser tube make it more suitable than a standard endotracheal tube when using a laser in the airway? (2 marks)

b) What other anaesthetic precautions should be taken when using a laser for airway surgery? (4 marks)

c) What should you do if an airway fire occurs? (3 marks)

d) Why are laser tubes not used for surgery other than airway surgery? (2 marks)

e) Describe an alternative method of airway management for laser surgery to the airway. (2 marks)

f) Name 4 precautions for staff protection that may be taken in the operating theatre when using lasers. (4 marks)

g) What does LASER stand for? (1 mark)

h) Name two types of laser commonly used in the operating theatre. (2 marks)

Answers

a) What features of a laser tube make it more suitable than a standard endotracheal tube when using a laser in the airway? (2 marks)
   - The metal is laser resistant, meaning that the tube is less likely to ignite and cause an airway fire

b) What other anaesthetic precautions should be taken when using a laser for airway surgery? (4 marks)
   - Avoid nitrous oxide
   - Use a low FiO_2 (ideally 21%)
   - Fill the cuff with water, rather than air
   - Protect other surfaces with wet swabs

c) What should you do if an airway fire occurs? (3 marks)
   - Switch the laser off
   - Flood the site of the fire with water
   - Disconnect the circuit and remove the endotracheal tube

d) Why are laser tubes not used for surgery other than airway surgery? (2 marks)
   - Expensive
   - Large external diameter with respect to a standard tube of the same internal diameter, making airway trauma more likely

e) Describe an alternative method of airway management for laser surgery to the airway. (2 marks)
   - Avoid intubation by using high frequency jet ventilation or insufflation. This removes the potential 'fuel' and reduces the risk of airway fire

f) Name 4 precautions for staff protection that may be taken in the operating theatre when using lasers. (4 marks)
   - Signs on external doors indicating that a laser is in use
   - Lock external doors so other staff cannot inadvertently walk in
   - Appropriate goggles for operating theatre staff
   - Cover windows

g) What does LASER stand for? (1 mark)
   - Light Amplification by Stimulated Emission of Radiation

h) Name two types of laser commonly used in the operating theatre. (2 marks)

   Any 2 of:
   - CO_2
   - Argon
   - NdYAG

7. Needlestick injury

Questions

a) Name 2 examples of personal protective equipment. (2 marks)

b) What should you do immediately following a needlestick injury? (3 marks)

c) Who should you report it to? (2 marks)

d) What should Occupational Health do? (1 mark)

e) Does a patient need to give consent for their blood to be tested following a needlestick injury to a healthcare professional? (1 mark)

f) What viruses should the patient's blood be tested for? (3 marks)

g) What types of injury increase the risk of a needlestick? (3 marks)

h) What are the percentage risks of seroconversion following a needlestick from a patient with: Hep B, Hep C, HIV? (3 marks)

i) Who does the NHS need to inform if a healthcare worker becomes infected following a needle stick injury? (1 mark)

j) By what percentage does post-exposure prophylaxis reduce the risk of seroconversion? (1 mark)

Answers

a) Name 2 examples of personal protective equipment. (2 marks)
- Gloves
- Goggles

b) What should you do immediately following a needle stick injury? (3 marks)
- Encourage the wound to bleed
- Wash with soap and running water
- Dry and cover the wound

c) Who should you report it to? (2 marks)
- Occupational Health Department OR
- Accident and Emergency if it occurs out of hours

d) What should Occupational Health do? (1 mark)
- Assess the risk of the injury to the health of the healthcare worker

e) Does a patient need to give consent for their blood to be tested following a needlestick injury to a healthcare professional? (1 mark)
- Yes

f) What viruses should the patient's blood be tested for? (3 marks)
- HIV
- Hepatitis B
- Hepatitis C

g) What types of injury increase the risk of a needlestick? (3 marks)

Any 3 of:
- Hollow needle
- Deep, muscular injuries
- Visible contamination of the needle with blood
- Procedure involved placing the device in an artery or vein

h) What are the percentage risks of seroconversion following a needlestick from a patient with: Hep B, Hep C, HIV? (3 marks)
- Hep B – 30% risk
- Hep C – 3% risk
- HIV – 0.3% risk

i) Who does the NHS need to inform if a healthcare worker becomes infected following a needle stick injury? (1 mark)
- Health Protection Agency

j) By what percentage does post-exposure prophylaxis reduce the risk of seroconversion? (1 mark)
- 80%

8. Peripheral nerve injury

Questions

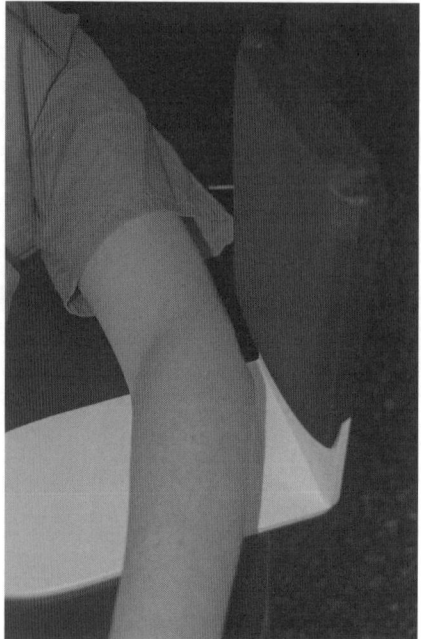

Figure 8.4 Position 1

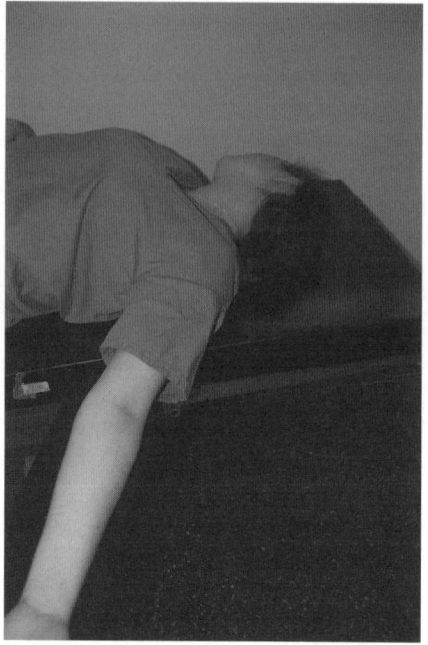

Figure 8.5 Position 2

a) Name 3 patient factors that make patients susceptible to perioperative nerve damage? (3 marks)
b) Name 3 anaesthetic factors that make patients susceptible to nerve damage? (3 marks)
c) What are the mechanisms by which peripheral nerves may be damaged? (3 marks)
d) Which nerve is at risk of damage in Figure 8.4? (1 mark)
e) What motor deficit will damage to this nerve cause? (3 marks)
f) What sensory deficit will damage to this nerve cause? (2 marks)
g) Which nerves are at risk of damage to a patient in the lithotomy position? (3 marks)
h) What is incorrect about the positioning of the patient in figure 8.5 and what type of injury might this cause? (2 marks)

Answers

a) Name 3 patient factors that make patients susceptible to perioperative nerve damage? (3 marks)

Any 3 of:
- Age – older patients are more at risk of nerve damage
- BMI – high and low
- Diabetes
- Rheumatoid arthritis

b) Name 3 anaesthetic factors that make patients susceptible to nerve damage? (3 marks)

Any 3 of:
- Long procedure
- Hypotension
- Hypoxia
- Hypovolaemia
- Prone or lithotomy position

c) What are the mechanisms by which peripheral nerves may be damaged? (3 marks)
- Direct damage
- Compression
- Angulation or strain

d) Which nerve is at risk of damage in Figure 8.4? (1 mark)
- Ulnar nerve

e) What motor deficit will damage to this nerve cause? (3 marks)
- Weak finger abduction and adduction
- Weak thumb adduction
- Weak flexion of medial 2 fingers

f) What sensory deficit will damage to this nerve cause? (2 marks)
- Sensory loss of medial hand and medial 1.5 fingers

g) Which nerves are at risk of damage to a patient in the lithotomy position? (3 marks)
- Sciatic (traction)
- Common peroneal (direct pressure)
- Obturator (traction)

h) What is incorrect about the positioning of the patient in figure 8.5 and what type of injury might this cause? (2 marks)
- Head should be neutral rather than turned away from the abducted arm
- Turning the head puts strain on the brachial plexus

9. Sterilisation

Questions

a) What is the Spaulding classification? (2 marks)

b) What is meant by 'critical items' with respect to infection risk? (2 marks)

c) What is meant by 'semi-critical' items? (2 marks)

d) Give examples of two items of anaesthetic equipment that are semi-critical. (2 marks)

e) What is decontamination? (1 mark)

f) What is disinfection? (1 mark)

g) What is a disinfectant? (1 mark)

h) Name 2 disinfectants with sporicidal activity. (2 marks)

i) What is meant by sterilisation? (1 mark)

j) What is the most common mode of sterilisation in hospital equipment? (1 mark)

k) Name 2 advantages of this mode of sterilization. (2 marks)

l) What 2 factors affect the efficacy of this process? (2 marks)

m) Which sterilisation modes are effective against prions? (1 mark)

Answers

a) What is the Spaulding classification? (2 marks)
- Classification that divides all hospital equipment into three categories based on risk of infection associated with its use
- Classifies equipment into critical, semi-critical and non-critical items

b) What is meant by 'critical items' with respect to infection risk? (2 marks)
- Items which enter the vasculature or other sterile tissues
- Examples include surgical instruments, central venous catheters and urinary catheters

c) What is meant by 'semi-critical' items? (2 marks)
- Items which contact mucous membranes and non-intact skin, but would not be expected to breach the blood stream
- They present an intermediate risk of infection

d) Give examples of two items of anaesthetic equipment that are semi-critical. (2 marks)

Any 2 of:
- Laryngoscopes
- Fibreoptic endoscopes
- Breathing circuits

e) What is decontamination? (1 mark)
- This describes the combination of cleaning, disinfection and/or sterilisation, which will render the item safe for further use

f) What is disinfection? (1 mark)
- A process which eliminates many or all pathologic organisms except spores

g) What is a disinfectant? (1 mark)
- A chemical agent used to disinfect inanimate objects (a chemical used to disinfect the body is called an antiseptic)

h) Name 2 disinfectants with sporicidal activity (2 marks)

Any 2 of:
- Peracetic acid
- Chlorine releasing agents e.g. sodium hypochorite
- Gluteraldehyde 2%

i) What is meant by sterilisation? (1 mark)
- A process which renders an object free of all viable infective organisms

j) What is the most common mode of sterilisation in hospital equipment? (1 mark)
- Steam sterilization

k) Name 2 advantages of this mode of sterilisation (2 marks)

Any 2 of:
- Non-toxic
- Non-corrosive
- Rapid
- Organisms are killed at a lower temperature using wet rather than dry heat

l) What 2 factors affect the efficacy of this process? (2 marks)
- Temperature
- Duration of exposure

m) Which sterilisation modes are effective against prions? (1 mark)
- None. It is thought that standard washing reduces the concentration exponentially with each cycle thus they are diminished to negligible levels

Further reading

Boumphrey S, Langton J. Electrical safety in the operating theatre. *Contin Educ Anaesth Crit Care Pain* 3 (1): 10– 14, 2003

Cross M, Plunkett E. *Physics, Pharmacology and Physiology for Anaesthetists*, Cambridge University Press, 2008

Maxwell MJ, Wilson MJ. Complications of blood transfusion. *Contin Educ Anaesth Crit Care Pain*, 6 (6): 225– 9, 2006

NHS Choices What should I do if I injure myself with a used needle? Available from http://www.nhs.uk/chq/Pages/2557.aspx?CategoryID=72

NHS Employers, Needlestick Injury. Available from http://www.nhsemployers.org/Aboutus/Publications/Documents/Needlestick%20injury.pdf Accessed January 2014

The Royal College of Anaesthetists. Hazards of positioning and pressure areas. e-Learning for Health, 2012

Sabir N, Ramachandra V. Decontamination of anaesthetic equipment. *Contin Educ Anaesth Crit Care Pain*, 4 (4): 103– 106, 2004

Serious Hazards of Transfusion, SHOT Report, (2012). Available from http://www.shotuk.org/wp-content/uploads/2013/08/SHOT-Annual-Report-2012.pdf

Singh S, Ingham R, Golding J. Basics of electricity for anaesthetists. *Contin Educ Anaesth Crit Care Pain*, 11 (6): 224– 8, 2011 www.wash-hands.com

World Health Organisation, Five Moments for Hand Hygiene. Available at http://www.who.int/gpsc/tools/Five_moments/en/

UK Blood Transfusion Service Handbook of Transfusion Medicine 2007. http://www.transfusionguidelines.org.uk/index.aspx?Publication=HTM

Chapter 9 **Measurement and Monitoring**

Introduction

Measurement and monitoring stations test basic science knowledge and focus on your understanding of principles, limitations, error and application. The station will often have a measurement or monitoring device to refer to, or a diagram or photograph of one.

There is some overlap with the physics questions in the Structured Oral Exam (SOE), but in the OSCE the questions tend to be more focused on practical applications. Measurement or monitoring questions will account for two of your OSCE stations.

1. Arterial line

Questions

Table 9.1 A list of incorrect ways that an arterial line can be set up

Incorrect Feature	Problem	Correction
5% Glucose for transduction		
Deflated pressure bag		
Venous cannula		
Venous line tubing		
Bubbles in line		
Transducer at the level of the patient's ear		

a) In Table 9.1, identify the problem with the errors listed in an arterial line set up and how these could be corrected. (6 marks)

b) How do you 'zero' an arterial line? (2 marks)

c) Why do we 'zero' arterial lines? (1 mark)

d) What is a pressure transducer? (1 mark)

e) How does a strain gauge work? (2 marks)

f) What information can you determine or derive from the arterial wave form? (4 marks)

g) What is damping? (1 mark)

h) List three features of an over damped arterial waveform? (2 marks)

i) What is optimal damping? (1 mark)

Answers

a) In Table 9.1, identify the problem with the errors listed in an arterial line set up and how these could be corrected. (6 marks)

Table 9.2 Table 9.2 Identify the problem with the errors listed in an arterial line set up and how these could be corrected

Incorrect Feature	Problem	Correction
5% Glucose for transduction	Infection risk	Normal saline (500ml) for transduction
Deflated pressure bag	Back flow of arterial blood, risk of clotting	Pressure bag to be maintained at 300mmHg
Venous cannula	Cannula is too long, compliant and will reduce the natural frequency	Appropriate arterial cannula
Venous line tubing	Tubing is too long and compliant thereby altering the natural frequency of the system	Specialised arterial line tubing
Bubbles in line	Damping, risk of air embolism	Purge line of air before connecting to patient
Transducer at the level of the patient's ear	Error in readings – elevation (7.5mmHg/ 10cm)	Lower transducer to level with the right atrium

b) Identify the problem with the errors listed in an arterial line set up and how these could be corrected?

c) How do you 'zero' an arterial line? (2 marks)
   • Open the 3-way tap to atmospheric pressure (not air), at level of right atrium (reference point at the level of the midaxillary line)

d) Why do we 'zero' arterial lines? (1 mark)
   • To ensure an accurate arterial pressure is obtained and to prevent baseline drift of the electrical circuits

e) What is a pressure transducer? (1 mark)
   • A transducer is a device that converts energy from one form into another. A pressure transducer changes pressure to electrical resistance or capacitance

f) How does a strain gauge work? (2 marks)
   • A strain gauge is a pressure transducer. Movement of a diaphragm occurs with changes in pressure which in turn alters the tension of a resistance wire. The change in resistance of the wire alters the current flow through a resistor

g) What information can you determine or derive from the arterial wave form? (4 marks)
   • Myocardial contractility – the rate of the rise of the upstroke (dp/dt)
   • Systemic vascular resistance – the position of the dicrotic notch and the rate of the down stroke
   • Stroke volume – area under curve from the start of the upstroke to the dicrotic notch
   • Cardiac output = heart rate x stroke volume

h) What is damping? (1 mark)
   • A dissipation of stored energy leading to a reduction in the amplitude of the oscillations

i) List three features of an over damped arterial waveform? (2 marks)
   • Narrowed pulse pressure (underestimation of systolic and overestimation of diastolic)
   • Slurred upstroke
   • Loss of dicrotic notch

j) What is optimal damping? (1 mark)
   • When there is a damping co-efficient of 0.64 (0.6–0.7). This results in the ideal arterial trace – a balance between rapid response to change and minimal overshoot

2. Temperature measurement

Questions

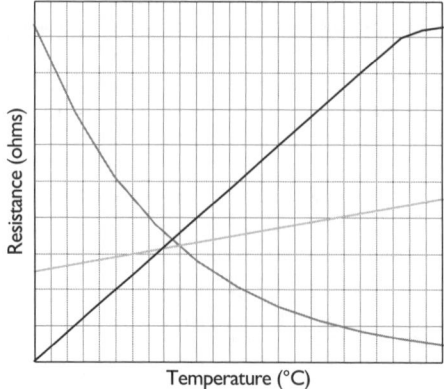

Figure 9.1 Graph. Please see colour plate section.

a) What is core temperature? (1 mark)
b) Name five ways that the body loses heat in theatre. (2 marks)
c) Name and define the SI unit of temperature measurement. (2 marks)
d) List three non-electrical and three electrical methods of measuring temperature. (3 marks)
e) Figure 9.1 represents electrical methods of temperature measurement. Identify and briefly describe their mechanism of action. State one advantage and disadvantage of each. (10 marks)
   (i)   Identify the blue line
   (ii) Identify the green line
   (iii) Identify the red line

Answers

a) What is core temperature? (1 mark)

- It is the operating temperature of the body and can be measured via oesophageal, bladder or tympanic routes in theatre
- It is tightly controlled at 37°C +/− 0.2°C by the hypothalamus in order to achieve optimum conditions for enzymatic reactions

b) Name five ways that the body loses heat in theatre. (2 marks)

- Radiation
- Convection
- Evaporation
- Conduction
- Respiration

c) Name and define the SI unit of temperature measurement. (2 marks)

- Kelvin
- 1 Kelvin = 1/273.16 of the thermodynamic triple point of water
- Temp (K) = temp (°C) + 273.15

d) List three non-electrical and three electrical methods of measuring temperature. (3 marks)

Non electrical
- Mercury thermometer
- Alcohol thermometer
- Bimetallic strip
- Bourdon gauge

Electrical
- Resistance wire
- Thermistor
- Thermocouple
- Infrared tympanic thermometer – thermopile (more than one thermocouple)

e) Figure 9.1 represents electrical methods of temperature measurement. Identify and briefly describe their mechanism of action. State one advantage and disadvantage of each. (10 marks)

- Identify the blue line: Thermistor
  - Mechanism of action: resistance of metal oxide semi-conductor falls as exponentially as temperature increase
  - Advantage: small, cheap, fast responding
  - Disadvantage: calibration errors (particularly in extreme temperatures), deteriorates over time
- Identify the green line: resistance wire
  - Mechanism of action: Resistance of a thin piece of metal increases with an increase in temperature (classically, platinum wire)
  - Advantage: simple
- Disadvantage: Expensive, insensitive Identify the red line: thermocouple
  - Mechanism of action: uses the Seebeck effect. The Seebeck effect describes the phenomenon where a voltage is produced at the junction of two dissimilar metals the magnitude of which is determined by the temperature difference between them. A second junction is required to complete the electrical circuit. It should be kept at a constant temperature
  - Advantage: fast response, accurate, can make small probes
  - Disadvantage: output voltage is small and signal amplification is often required

3. Mono-auricular stethoscope

Questions

This question is about mono-auricular stethoscopes.

a) List 2 indications for use? (2 marks)
b) What is an air embolism, and what volumes are significant? (2 marks)
c) Name two factors that determine the effect of the venous air embolism? (2 marks)
d) List five surgical procedures that predispose to air embolism. (5 marks)
e) List the clinical features of air embolism. (4 marks)
f) Name 2 other devices that can be used to detect air embolism? (2 marks)
g) Briefly outline the management of air embolism. (3 marks)

Answers

This question is about mono-auricular stethoscopes.

a) List 2 indications for use. (2 marks)
- Continuous auscultation of breath and heart sounds; traditionally used in paediatric surgery
- Surgery with a high risk of air embolism e.g. neurosurgery; posterior fossa surgery, sitting craniotomies

b) What is an air embolism, and what volumes are significant? (2 marks)
- Entrainment of air from the operative field into the venous or arterial vasculature causing systemic effects
- 3–5 ml/kg is lethal but 0.5ml/kg will cause clinical effect

c) Name two factors that determine the effect of the venous air embolism. (2 marks)
- Rate of air accumulation
- Volume of air entrained

d) List five surgical procedures that predispose to air embolism. (3 marks)
- Neurosurgical procedures – sitting craniotomies, posterior fossa surgery, cervical laminectomy and spinal fusion surgeries
- Head and neck- thyroidectomy, radical neck dissection, eye surgery
- Cardiothoracic – cardiac air embolism, blast injuries, open chest wounds
- Orthopaedic – hip replacement, arthroscopy, shoulder surgery in sitting position
- General – laparoscopic cholecystectomy, liver transplants, prostatectomies
- Obstetrics and gynaecology – caesarean section, laparoscopic surgery

e) List the clinical features of air embolism. (5 marks)
- Respiratory: fall in oxygen saturations, wheeze, fall in end tidal CO_2
- Cardiovascular: cardiac output falls, eventually leading to cardiovascular collapse. Other features may be present including:
  - Tachyarrythmias
  - Pulmonary hypertension
  - Right heart failure (raised JVP)
  - ST changes and peaked T waves
  - Chest pain
  - Mill wheel murmur
- Neurological: altered mental state

f) Name 2 other devices that can be used to detect air embolism. (2 marks)
- Echocardiography – TOE or TTE
- Pulmonary artery catheter
- Precordial doppler

g) Briefly outline the management of air embolism. (3 marks)
- Inform theatre team that a critical incident has occurred
- Call for help
- Start CPR if appropriate
  - Compressions may break up the 'air lock' and improve situation
- Prevent further air entrainment by: informing surgeons to flood field with saline, compress wound site.

- Discontinue nitrous oxide
- Increase venous pressure
- Airway and breathing: ensure airway is secure, FIO2 1.0, IPPV with PEEP
- Circulation: reduce cardiovascular impact by moving the patient into the left decubitus position, instigate cardiovascular support using IV fluids and inotropes
- Attempt to aspirate air from any CVP line (if present).

4. Wright's respirometer

Questions

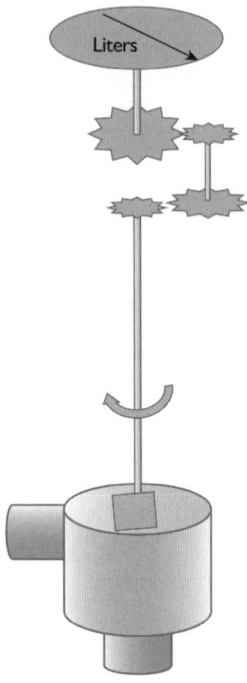

Figure 9.2 Measuring equipment

a) What is Figure 9.2 a diagram of? (2 marks)
b) What does it measure? (2 marks)
c) What variable can be calculated? (2 marks)
d) How does it work? (3 marks)
e) In a ventilated patient where would you position it in the patient circuit and why? (2 marks)
f) When is it inaccurate, give three examples? (3 marks)
g) Name 2 advantages of this device? (2 marks)
h) How does it differ from a pneumotachograph? (2 marks)
i) How does a pneumotachograph work? (2 marks)

Answers

a) What is Figure 9.2 a diagram of? (2 marks)
- Wright's respirometer

b) What does it measure? (2 marks)
- Gas volume

c) What variable can be calculated? (2 marks)
- Gas flow – average recorded volume over a period of time

d) How does it work? (3 marks)
- Allows gas flow in one direction only (unidirectional)
- The slits create a circular flow to rotate the vane (150 revolutions for each litre of gas)
- The pointer demonstrates the volume

e) In a ventilated patient where would you position it in the patient circuit and why? (2 marks)
- Where? Expiratory limb (lower pressure than inspiratory) and as close to the patient as possible
- Why? To minimise the loss of gas due to expansion of tubing and leaks

   Accuracy is 5–10%.

f) When is it inaccurate? Give three examples. (3 marks)
- Under-reads at low volumes (less than 2L)
- Over-reads at high volumes
- Water condensation may cause pointer to stick

g) Name 2 advantages of this device? (2 marks)
- No power source required
- Lightweight and therefore portable

h) How does it differ from a pneumotachograph? (2 marks)
- A pneumotachograph measures flow not volume (though flow can be calculated from a respirometer)

i) How does a pneumotachograph work? (2 marks)
- It measures a pressure change across a fixed resistance, and flow can be calculated according to Ohm's law
- Pressure transducers measure the pressure on either side of a gauze. The gauze is large enough to permit laminar flow

5. Humidity

Questions

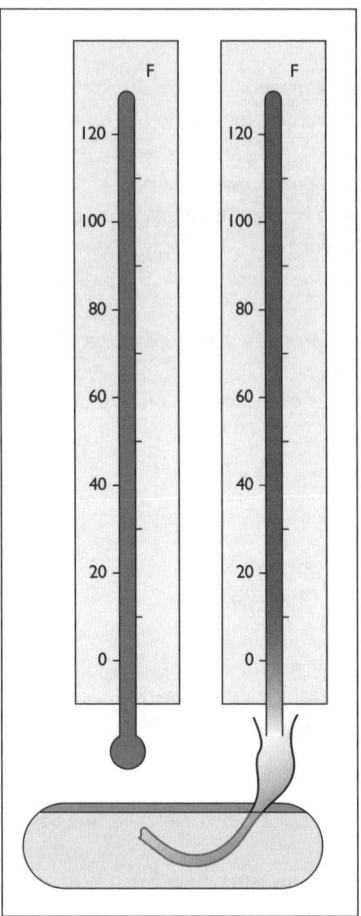

Figure 9.3 Hygrometer

a) What is definition of absolute humidity? (1 mark)
b) What units is absolute humidity measured in? (1 mark)
c) What is definition of relative humidity? (2 marks)
d) Name the equipment shown in Figure 9.3. (1 mark)
e) How does the equipment in Figure 9.3 work? (4 marks)
f) What piece of equipment used for measuring humidity uses the dew point and what is the dew point? (2 marks)
g) What does a hair hygrometer measure and how? (3 marks)
h) What is the absolute humidity of fully saturated air at 37°C? (1 mark)
i) What is the recommended humidity in theatre and why should it be kept at this level? (3 mark)
j) List four methods employed to provide humidification. (2 marks)

Answers

a) What is definition of absolute humidity? (1 mark)
- Mass of water vapour in given volume of air

b) What units is absolute humidity measured in? (1 mark)
- g/m^3 or mglL

c) What is definition of relative humidity? (2 marks)
- Ratio of mass of water vapour in given volume of air to mass required to saturate given volume at same temperature (expressed as percentage)

d) Name the equipment shown in Figure 9.3. (1 mark)
- Wet and dry hygrometer

e) How does the equipment in Figure 9.3 work? (4 marks)
- The wet and dry hygrometers measure relative humidity
- The dry bulb measures true ambient temperature
- The wet bulb measures a lower temperature because of the cooling effect from the evaporation of surrounding water and the loss of latent heat of vaporisation
- The temperature difference is related to the rate of evaporation which is determined by the ambient humidity
- The relative humidity can then be determined by referencing the temperature difference on pre-calculated tables

f) What piece of equipment used for measuring humidity uses the dew point and what is the dew point? (2 marks)
- Regnault's hygrometer
- The dew point is the temperature at which ambient air is saturated with water vapour and condenses on a cold surface to form 'dew'

g) What does a hair hygrometer measure and how? (3 marks)
- What? Relative humidity
- How! As humidity increases the hair gets longer, moving a pointer along a scale which can be read

h) What is the absolute humidity of fully saturated air at 37°C? (1 mark)
- $44g/m^3$

i) What is the recommended humidity in theatre and why should it be kept at this level? (3 mark)
- Humidity Relative humidity of 30–60%
- Why: low humidity environments can lead to the spread and proliferation of contaminants and can lead to mucosal dryness, affecting the respiratory system, eyes and skin. It can contribute to the build-up of static. High humidity can be uncomfortable for staff

j) List four methods employed to provide humidification. (2 marks)
- HME (heat and moisture exchange) filters
- Nebulisers
- Hot water bath humidifiers
- Soda lime

6. Carbon dioxide measurement

Questions

a) What is a capnograph? (1 mark)

b) What is an infrared analyser? (2 marks)

c) Carbon dioxide absorbs infrared radiation at what wavelength? (1 mark)

d) What is the collision broadening effect? (2 marks)

e) What is the sample chamber window made from and why? (1 mark)

f) List two types of infrared capnograph and four differences between them in Table 9.3. (5 marks)

Table 9.3 Types of capnograph

Type of capnograph
Difference 1
Difference 2
Difference 3
Difference 4

g) List five ways to measure carbon dioxide. (5 marks)

h) List three pieces of information with clinical significance that can be obtained from a capnograh trace. (3 marks)

Answers

a) What is a capnograph? (1 mark)
  - An instrument which provides a continuous recording of carbon dioxide concentration
b) What is an infrared analyser? (2 marks)
  - Gases that have two or more dissimilar atoms will absorb radiation within the infrared spectrum. By measuring the absorbed fraction of radiation the partial pressure of the gas can be determined
  - The absorption bandwidth needs to be narrow to allow the analyser to differentiate between the gases
c) Carbon dioxide absorbs infrared radiation at what wavelength? (1 mark)
  - 4.25–4.3µm
d) What is the collision broadening effect? (2 marks)
  - A falsely high carbon dioxide reading may occur in the presence of nitrous oxide which absorbs infrared at a similar wavelength of 4.5µm
  - The carbon dioxide reading may also be affected by the proximity of nitrous oxide molecules, causing an alteration in energy that may broaden the infrared wavelength at which they are absorbed
e) What is the sample chamber window made from and why? (1 marks)
  - A material that is transparent to infrared radiation such as sapphire Glass absorbs infrared radiation
f) List two types of infrared capnograph and four differences between them in Table 9.3. (5 marks)
  - See the answers in Table 9.4.

Table 9.4 Types of capnograph

Type of capnography	Main stream analyser	Side stream analyser
Difference 1	Sample chamber is positioned within patient's circuit	Sample chamber is at a distant site connected to patient via an adaptor close to trachea using Teflon sampling tube
Difference 2	No lag time before gas reaches sample chamber	Lag time before gas reaches sample chamber (dependent on length and diameter of sample tube)
Difference 3	Multiple gases and vapours cannot be measured simultaneously	Can analyse multiple gases
Difference 4	Used on intubated patients	Can be used on self-ventilating, non-intubated patients

g) List five ways to measure carbon dioxide. (5 marks)
  - Severinghaus electrode
  - Infrared spectroscopy
  - Raman Scattering
  - Mass spectrometry
  - Colorimetry
  - Siggaard Anderson nomogram
h) List three pieces of information with clinical significance that can be obtained from a capnograh trace. (3 marks)
  - End tidal carbon dioxide: rebreathing, hypoventilation, hyperventilation
  - Waveform: neuromuscular blocker wearing off, airway obstruction (COPD, compression of tube), disconnections
  - Cardiac output

7. ECG

Questions

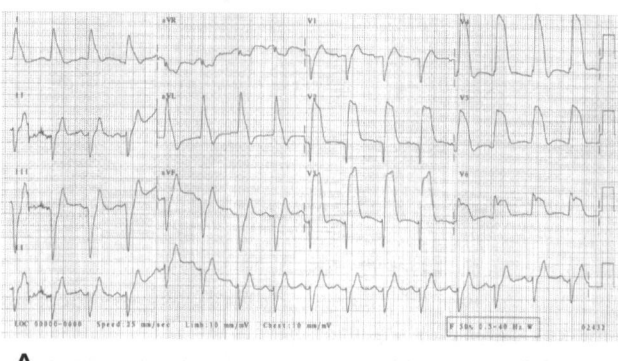

A

Figure 9.4a ECG

Reproduced from Myerson SG et al., *Emergencies in Cardiology*, copyright 2009 with permission from Oxford University Press

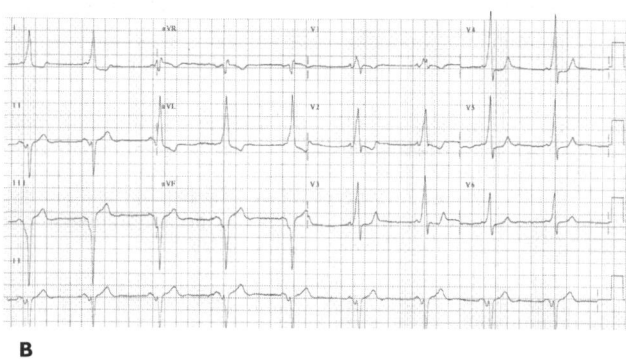

B

Figure 9.4b ECG

Reproduced from Myerson SG et al., *Emergencies in Cardiology*, copyright 2009 with permission from Oxford University Press

Look at Figure 9.4a.

a) At what speed are ECGs usually recorded? (1 mark)
b) What is the heart rate shown above? (1 mark)
c) Is there left axis deviation? (1 mark)
d) What is the abnormality? (1 mark)
e) What is the diagnosis? (1 mark)
f) Which blood vessel is likely to be occluded? (2 marks)
g) List three ECG abnormalities that may be present in a patient with a pulmonary embolus. (3 marks)

Look at Figure 9.4b.

h) What is the axis? (1 mark)

i) What is the normal PR interval? (1 mark)

j) What is the P wave abnormality shown in leads II and III? (2 marks)

k) What is the diagnosis and underlying problem? (2 marks)

l) Would digoxin be a likely first-line therapy? (2 marks)

m) What is bifascicular block? (2 marks)

Answers

a) At what speed are ECGs usually recorded? (1 mark)
- 25mm per second

b) What is the heart rate shown above? (1 mark)
- 100 beats per minute (one large square on the ECG recording represents 0.2 s and 300 large squares represent one minute)

c) Is there left axis deviation? (1 mark)
- No

d) What is the abnormality? (1 mark)
- ST elevation in leads V1–V3, Lead I and aVL

e) What is the diagnosis? (1 mark)
- Acute anterolateral myocardial infarction

f) Where would the likely site of occlusion be on a coronary angiogram? (2 marks)
- The left anterior descending artery +/− circumflex artery

g) List three ECG abnormalities that may be present in a patient with a pulmonary embolus. (3 marks)
- Peaked P waves
- Deep S waves in I (right axis deviation)
- Tall R waves in V1
- Right bundle branch block
- Inverted T waves in leads V2, V3
- Pathological 'Q' wave in lead III
- Inverted T waves in lead III
- Atrial fibrillation

Remember mnemonic 'SI, QIII, TIII', which is uncommonly seen, but refers to deep S waves in lead I, pathological Q wave in Lead III and inverted T waves in lead III.
Look at Figure 9.4b.

h) What is the axis? (1 mark)
- Normal axis. QRS complexes predominantly positive in leads I and III

i) What is the normal PR interval? (1 mark)
- 0.12–0.2 seconds

j) What is the P wave abnormality shown in leads II and III? (1 mark)
- Shortened PR interval.
- Characteristic delta waves – slurred upslope of the R wave due to the shortened PR interval

k) What is the diagnosis and underlying problem? (2 marks)
- Wolff-Parkinson-White syndrome
- An accessory pathway is present between the atria and ventricle which causes early depolarisation

l) Would digoxin be a likely first-line therapy? (2 marks)
- No
- Digoxin is contra-indicated as it slows conduction at the AV node, thereby facilitating conduction via the accessory pathway

m) What is bifascicular block? (2 marks)
- Right bundle branch block and left axis deviation
- Indicates widespread damage to the conducting system, with blockage of the right bundle branch and the left anterior fascicle

8. Oxygen measurement

Questions

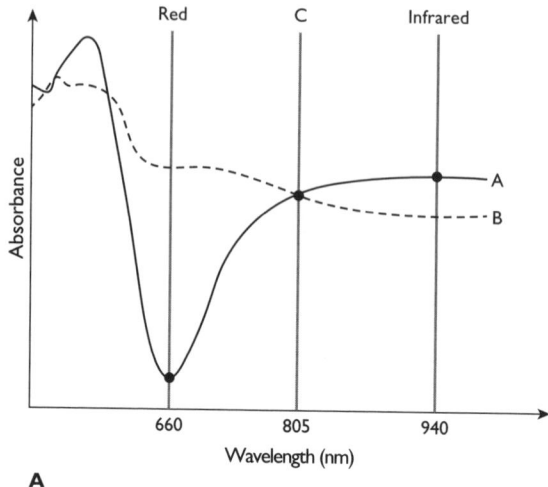

Figure 9.5a Absorbance spectra

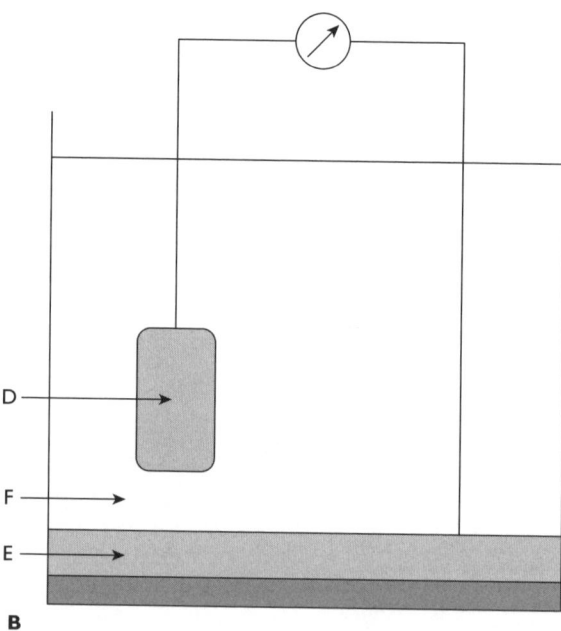

Figure 9.5b Fuel cell. Please see colour plate section.

a) State Lambert's Law. (1 mark)
b) What, in nanometres, are the two wavelengths of the light sources in a pulse oximeter? (2 marks)

Look at Figure 9.5a

c) What, in relation to pulse oximetry, do A and B represent? (1 mark)
d) What is C? (2 marks)
e) Give two situations where readings from a pulse oximeter may not be accurate. (2 marks)

Look at Figure 9.5b

f) Concerning measurement of the concentration of oxygen in a gas mixture, what equipment does Figure 9.5b represent? (1 mark)
g) Name the labelled parts D, E, and F. (3 marks)
h) What happens to oxygen molecules as they diffuse through the membrane? (2 marks)
i) Does the above equipment require a battery? (1 mark)
j) Why does this equipment need a thermistor? (1 mark)
k) What happens when oxygen is added? (1 mark)
l) What gives oxygen its paramagnetic property? (2 marks)
m) Name one other method, aside from those discussed above, of measuring the concentration of oxygen in a gas mixture. (1 mark)

Answers

a) State Lambert's Law. (1 mark)
- The absorption of radiation by a solution is directly proportional to the thickness of the absorbing layer

b) What, in nanometres, are the two wavelengths of the light sources in a pulse oximeter? (2 marks)
- 660nm (visible red spectrum)
- 940nm (infrared spectrum)

Look at Figure 9.5a

c) What, in relation to pulse oximetry, do A and B represent? (2 marks)
- A – absorbance spectrum of oxyhaemoglobin
- B – absorbance spectrum of deoxyhaemoglobin

d) What is C? (2 marks)
- Isobestic point
- Point where the absorbance of the two forms of haemoglobin is equal

e) Give two situations where readings from a pulse oximeter may not be accurate. (2 marks)
- Abnormal haemoglobins (methaemoglobin, carboxyhaemoglobin)
- Peripheral vasoconstriction (peripheral vascular disease, shock)
- Venous pulsation or congestion such as in tricuspid regurgitation
- External disturbances e.g. diathermy, shivering, nail polish

Look at Figure 9.5b

f) Concerning measurement of the concentration of oxygen in a gas mixture, what equipment does Figure 9.5b represent? (1 mark)
- A galvanic fuel cell

g) Name the labelled parts D, E, and F. (3 marks)
- D – Lead anode
- E – Gold cathode
- F – Potassium hydroxide solution

h) What happens to oxygen molecules as they diffuse through the membrane? (2 marks)
- Combine with the electrons and water at the cathode to form hydroxyl ions

i) Does the above equipment require a battery? (1 mark)
- No – the fuel cell produces a voltage and so acts as a battery

j) Why does this equipment need a thermistor? (1 mark)
- This allows temperature compensation to help maintain fuel cell output

With respect to a simple paramagnetic oxygen analyser in a non-uniform magnetic field

k) What happens when oxygen is added? (2 marks)
- The oxygen is attracted into the magnetic field and will displace the glass spheres, so rotating the dumb-bell

l) What gives oxygen its paramagnetic property? (2 marks)
- The electrons in the outer shell of the oxygen molecule are unpaired

m) Name one other method, aside from those discussed above, of measuring the concentration of oxygen in a gas mixture. (1 mark)
- Mass spectrometry
- Oxygen electrode

9. Nerve stimulators

Questions

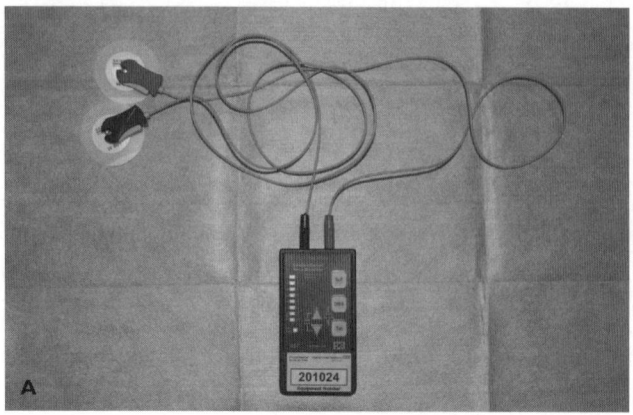

Figure 9.6a Equipment to stimulate nerves. Please see colour plate section.

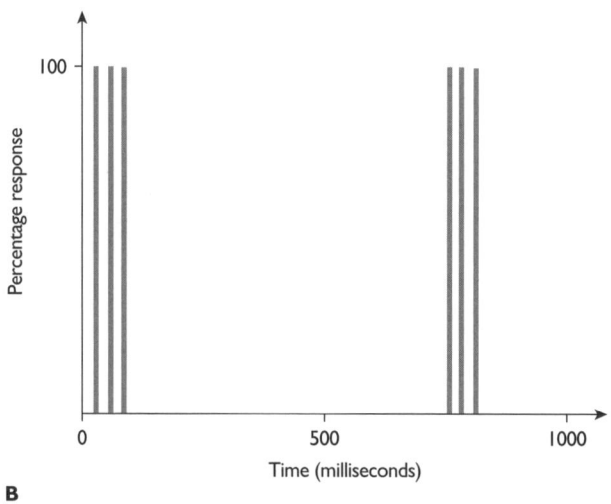

Figure 9.6b Graph

a) What is Figure 9.6a? (1 mark)
b) Describe where you would place the positive and negative electrodes for stimulating the ulnar nerve. (2 marks)
c) What response would you observe when the ulnar nerve is stimulated? (2 marks)
d) Name two other peripheral nerves that may be used for monitoring purposes. (2 marks)
e) What peak current is typically delivered by the equipment shown? (1 mark)
f) What type of stimulation is shown in the Figure 9.6b and what does it comprise? (3 marks)

g) What response to this type of stimulation is seen in a partially paralysed patient? (2 marks)

h) What is a 'train-of-four' stimulus? (2 marks)

i) What is the 'train-of-four count' or 'train-of-four ratio'? (1 mark)

j) During non-depolarising blockade, at what percentage acetylcholine receptor occupancy will the fourth twitch height start to decrease? (1 mark)

k) When assessed mechanically, is double burst stimulation more sensitive than train-of-four? (2 marks)

l) Which type of muscle relaxants exhibit fade with a train-of-four stimulus? (1 mark)

Answers

a) What is Figure 9.6a? (1 mark)
- Peripheral nerve stimulator

b) Describe where you would place the positive and negative electrodes for stimulating the ulnar nerve. (2 marks)
- Negative electrode should be distal, 1cm proximal to the flexion crease of the wrist on the medial border of the forearm
- Positive electrode should be proximal, 2–3cm proximal to the distal electrode, also on the medial border of the forearm

c) What response would you observe when the ulnar nerve is stimulated? (2 marks)
- Contraction of adductor pollicis brevis (adduction of thumb)

d) Name two other peripheral nerves that may be used for monitoring purposes (2 marks)
- Common peroneal nerve at the neck of the fibula
- Posterior tibial nerve at the ankle
- Facial nerve

e) What peak current is typically delivered by the equipment shown? (1 mark)
- 60 mA

f) What type of stimulation is shown in the Figure 9.6b and what does it comprise? (3 marks)
- Double burst stimulation
- Comprises: two short bursts of 50Hz tetanic stimulation (3 x 0.2ms stimuli, separated by 20ms) separated by 750ms

g) What response to this type of stimulation is seen in a partially paralysed patient? (2 marks)
- The second muscle contraction is weaker than the first

h) What is a 'train-of-four' stimulus? (2 marks)
- Four stimuli delivered at 2Hz over 2 seconds

i) What is the 'train-of-four count' or 'train-of-four ratio'? (1 mark)
- The ratio of the strength of the fourth twitch to the first

j) During non-depolarising blockade, at what percentage acetylcholine receptor occupancy will the fourth twitch height start to decrease? (1 mark)
- 70–75%

k) When assessed mechanically, is double burst stimulation more sensitive than train-of-four? (2 marks)
- No
- Double burst stimulation was developed to allow easy manual detection of small amounts of residual neuromuscular blockade

l) Which type of muscle relaxants exhibit fade with a train-of-four stimulus? (1 mark)
- Non-depolarising muscle relaxants

10. Vaporisers

Questions

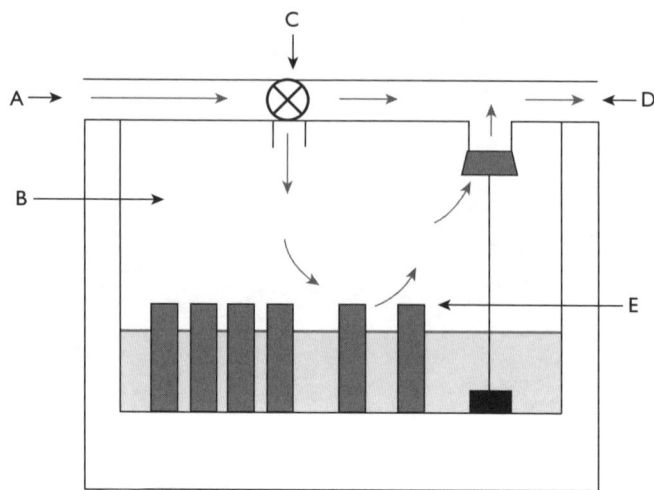

Figure 9.7 Vaporiser. Please see colour plate section.

a) What is a vaporiser? (2 marks)
b) Name three characteristics of the ideal vaporiser. (3 marks)
c) What type of vaporiser is shown in Figure 9.7? (1 mark)
d) Label the diagram. (4 marks)
e) What is C comprised of? (1 mark)
f) What is the function of C? (1 mark)
g) Why is C necessary? (2 marks)
h) One channel of gas is fully saturated with anaesthetic vapour before it rejoins the stream leaving the vaporiser. List two ways this can be achieved. (2 marks)
i) How does a Desflurane vaporiser differ from what has been discussed? (2 marks)
j) What happens to the percentage of vapour carried by the fresh gas flow at high altitudes? (1 mark)
k) Is this of clinical relevance? Why? (1 mark)

Answers

a) What is a vaporiser? (2 marks)
- A piece of equipment which allows a controlled amount of inhalational anaesthetic agent to be added to the fresh gas flow, after changing it from liquid to vapour form

b) Name three characteristics of the ideal vaporiser. (3 marks)
- Performance is not affected by changes in fresh gas flow, volume of liquid anaesthetic agent, ambient pressure and temperature, and decrease in temperature due to vaporisation
- Low resistance to flow
- Light weight
- Economical
- Hard-wearing construction, with resistance to corrosion and minimal servicing requirements

c) What type of vaporiser is shown in Figure 9.7? (1 mark)
- Plenum vaporiser

d) Label the diagram. (4 marks)
- A – fresh gas inlet
- B – vaporising chamber
- C – bimetallic strip
- D – bypass channel

e) What is C comprised of? (1 mark)
- Two strips of metal with different coefficients of thermal expansion joined together

f) What is the function of C? (1 mark)
- As the temperature changes, the shape of the strip alters. It acts as a temperature-sensitive valve controlling the splitting ratio of the gas flow

g) Why is C necessary? (2 marks)
- As the anaesthetic agent vaporises, it draws latent heat of vaporisation from the remaining anaesthetic liquid and from the walls of the vaporiser
- The temperature falls, as does the saturated vapour pressure of the anaesthetic agent
- Unless the splitting ratio of the fresh gas flow is altered, the concentration of anaesthetic vapour leaving the chamber would also fall
- The vaporiser would become inaccurate

h) One channel of gas is fully saturated with anaesthetic vapour before it rejoins the stream leaving the vaporiser. List two ways this can be achieved. (2 marks)
- The vaporising chamber contains wicks saturated by the inhalational agent
- The vaporising chamber contains a series of baffles
- The gas is bubbled through the anaesthetic liquid

All above measures are designed to increase the surface area of contact between the carrier gas and the anaesthetic agent.

i) How does a Desflurane vaporiser differ from what has been discussed? (2 marks)
- Desflurane has a boiling point of 22.6°C. This is close to usual 'room temperature', and so desflurane requires a special design of vaporiser for its use to ensure accurate vaporisation
- The desflurane is held in a chamber maintained at a temperature of 39°C

j) What happens to the percentage of vapour carried by the fresh gas flow at high altitudes? (1 mark)
- The percentage of vapour increases

k) Is this of clinical relevance? Why? (1 mark)

- No
- It is the partial pressure of the agent in the alveoli that determines the clinical effect of the anaesthetic agent

Further reading

Al-Shaikh B, Stacey S. *Essentials of Anaesthetic Equipment* (3rd edn). Churchill Livingstone, 138–42, 146–7, 162–4, 173–4, 2008

Davis P, Kenny G. *Basic Physics and Measurement in Anaesthesia* (5th edn). Butterworth Heinmann, 24–5, 33–4, 97–104, 192–96, 128–31, 213–18, 2007

Cross M, Plunkett E. *Physics, Pharmacology and Physiology for Anaesthetists*. Cambridge University Press, 30–2, 2008

Webber S, Andrzejowski J, Francis G. Gas Embolism in Anaesthesia. *BJA CEPD Reviews* 2 (2): 53–7, 2002

Chapter 10 **Resuscitation and Simulation**

Introduction

The purpose of this chapter is to act as a starting point for your revision for the resuscitation and simulation stations. There will be three of these stations in your exam; one interactive resuscitation, one resuscitation skills station and one simulation station.

These stations are practical stations and so are difficult to prepare for on your own solely using a revision text. This chapter is designed to take you through some of the typical scenarios that you might encounter and refresh the knowledge that you will be expected to be familiar with when at these stations.

Resuscitation and simulation stations will often be based on 2016 ALS guidelines, Difficult Airway Society Guidelines and The Association of Anaesthatists in Great Britain and Ireland (AAGBI) guidelines. It is worth familiarising yourself with the most important of these.

1. Narrow complex tachycardia

Questions

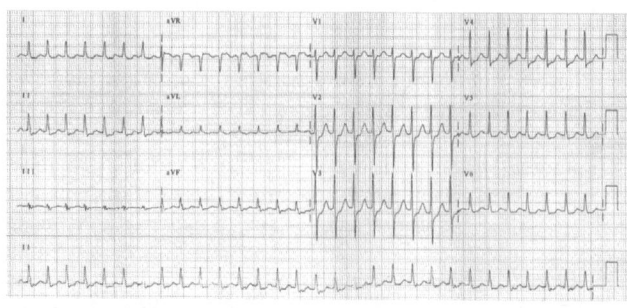

Figure 10.1 ECG

Reproduced from Myerson SG *et al. Emergencies in Cardiology*, 2009. With permission from Oxford University Press

Look at the ECG in Figure 10.1 and answer the following questions:

a) What does it show? (1 mark)
b) What is the Rate? (1 mark)
c) What is the Rhythm? (1 mark)
d) What is the QRS interval? (1 mark)

You are presented with this ECG and asked to review the patient that it belongs to.

e) What is your immediate management? (3 marks)
f) List the adverse clinical features associated with such an arrhythmia. (4 marks)
g) The patient demonstrates no adverse signs at this stage. How would you proceed with management of this patient? (3 marks)
h) Despite your intervention your patient becomes breathless, complains of chest pain and drops her blood pressure. How would you proceed? (4 marks)
i) With respect to synchronised direct current (DC) cardioversion; what energy level would you use? (2 marks)

Answers

a) What does it show? (1 mark)
- Narrow complex tachycardia, consistent with a supraventricular tachycardia

b) What is the Rate? (1 mark)
- 200bpm

c) What is the Rhythm? (1 mark)
- Regular

d) What is the QRS interval? (1 mark)
- Less than 0.12 s or 0.08 seconds

You are presented with this ECG and asked to review the patient that it belongs to.

e) What is your immediate management? (3 marks)
- Use an ABC approach
- Give high-flow oxygen
- Establish intravenous access
- Apply full monitoring- oxygen saturation, ECG recording, non-invasive blood pressure
- Look for reversible causes
- Identify any adverse signs (see below)

f) List the adverse clinical features associated with such an arrhythmia. (4 marks)
- Heart failure
- Myocardial ischaemia
- Shock
- Syncope

g) The patient demonstrates no adverse signs at this stage. How would you proceed with management of this patient? (3 marks)
- Ensure continuous ECG monitoring
- Vagal manoeuvres, unless contra-indicated
- Adenosine 6mg, 12mg, 12mg
- If adenosine is contraindicated or fails consider verapamil 2.5–5mg

h) Despite your intervention your patient becomes breathless, complains of chest pain and drops her blood pressure. How would you proceed? (4 marks)
- Call for help
- Provide patient with analgesia and sedation
- Deliver up to 3 synchronised DC shocks (70–120J)
- Amiodarone: 300mg intravenously over 10–20mins, followed by 900mg over 24 hours

i) With respect to synchronised DC cardioversion; what energy level would you use? (2 marks)
- For broad complex tachycardias or AF start at 120–150J biphasic (200J monophasic), increasing incrementally if this fails
- For atrial flutter or regular narrow complex tachycardia's start at 70–120J biphasic (100J monophasic) as these can usually be terminated with lower energy levels

2. Near drowning

Questions

You are called to the Emergency Department as part of the resuscitation team. The call is for a suspected drowning in a young adult. As you arrive, paramedics bring in the patient, and you notice that CPR is in progress.

a) What is your initial management? (5 marks)
b) What reversible causes would you look for? (4 marks)
c) Which are most likely in this case to be present? (4 marks)
d) The patient has a core temperature of 28°C. How does this alter your management? (4 marks)
e) Define mild, moderate and severe hypothermia. (3 marks)

Answers

a) What is your initial management? (5 marks)
- Ensure full resuscitation team is present
- Confirm cardiac arrest
- Provide basic airway support via bag-valve-mask and give high-flow oxygen
- Immobilise C-spine
- Safely transfer patient onto trolley (suspect other injuries) ensuring CPR is ongoing at a ratio of 30 compressions to 2 ventilations
- Attach defibrillator – shock if appropriate
- Take handover from the paramedics
- Secure airway early
- Establish IV access, give warmed fluids, take bloods and a blood gas
- Identify any reversible causes

b) What reversible causes would you look for? (4 marks)
- Hypoxia
- Hypothermia
- Hypo- or hyper-kalaemia/-magnesaemia/-calcaemia
- Hypovolaemia
- Thromboembolism
- Tamponade
- Tension pneumothorax
- Toxins

c) Which are most likely in this case to be present? (4 marks)
- Hypothermia
- Hypoxia
- Hypovolaemia
- Consider toxins or thromboembolism as a cause of collapse leading to drowning

d) The patient has a core temperature of 28°C. How does this alter your management? (4 marks)
- Secure airway early
- CPR should be continued until the patient is normothermic
- No more than 3 shocks should be given (if indicated) until the patient's temperature is >30°C
- No drugs should be administered until temperature is >30°C and then administer at double the normal interval (between doses) until normothermia is achieved
- Active rewarming – take off wet clothes, dry and cover patient with hot air blankets and increase ambient room temperature if possible. Warmed intravenous fluid and oxygen. Consider warmed fluid via NG tube and bladder catheter. Avoid hyperthermia on rewarming. Large amounts of iv fluids may be required as the patient rewarms and vasodilates
- Monitor electrolytes, glucose and blood gases carefully as they may alter rapidly with correction of hypothermia

e) Define mild, moderate and severe hypothermia. (3 marks)
- Hypothermia is described as a core body temperature of less than 35°C
  - Mild 32–35°C
  - Moderate 30–32°C
  - Severe <30°C

3. Anaesthetic emergency I

Questions

You are the solo anaesthetist for a gynaecology list. You induce anaesthesia without incident (in the anaesthetic room) in a fit and well 27-year-old woman for a laparoscopic procedure. When you take the patient through to theatre and attach her to the ventilator and monitor, you notice that she has high airway pressures, with oxygen saturations of 90%, a blood pressure of 60/30mmHg and a heart rate of 140bpm.

a) What do you do? (5 marks)

b) You notice a rash and bronchospasm is clearly audible. What treatment would you instigate (include doses)? (4 marks)

c) What investigations should be undertaken in this patient? (2 marks)

d) Who should be informed of event? (2 marks)

e) Define anaphylaxis? (1 mark)

f) What kind of hypersensitivity reactions occur to latex? (2 marks)

g) List 4 groups that are at increased risk of latex allergy? (4 marks)

Answers

a) What do you do? (5 marks)
- Call for help, note time
- Approach in an ABC manner
- Give 100% oxygen
- Check position of endotracheal tube, auscultate for bilateral air entry and bronchospasm
- Establish wide bore iv access (if not already done) and give fluids
- Lie patient flat and elevate legs
- Give vasopressors, consider adrenaline (if signs of anaphylaxis)
- Frequent observations (ECG, BP and saturations)
- Look for other causes; look for urticaria and check for equipment failure. This is probable anaphylaxis.
- Remove precipitating cause (consider muscle relaxant, antibiotics, gelofusin, latex, chlorhexidine as causes)
- Maintain anaesthesia

a) You notice a rash and bronchospasm is clearly audible. What treatment would you instigate (include doses)? (4 marks)
- Adrenaline 500mcg intramuscular injection (IM) or 50mcg IV, repeated as required
- Start an infusion if repeated doses are required.
- Chlorphenamine 10mg IV
- Hydrocortisone 200mg IV or IM
- IV fluid challenge 500–1000ml
- Crystalloid preferred as some colloids may precipitate anaphylaxis
- Salbutamol via endotracheal tube or IV if no inhaler or nebuliser available. Increase inhaled concentration of volatile to bronchodilate (if blood pressure permits) and consider magnesium sulphate
- Arrange critical care bed

b) What investigations should be undertaken in this patient? (2 marks)
- Mast cell tryptase
- Take at commencement of resuscitation, 1–2 hours post-event and 24 hours afterwards
- Consult allergy and immunology centre and give a detailed account of events, timings and drugs given
- Skin, intradermal and patch testing will be done in the allergy centre following complete recovery

c) Who should be informed of event? (2 marks)
- Patient and next of kin
- Patient's GP
- Allergy clinic

d) Define anaphylaxis? (1 mark)
- A severe life-threatening generalised or systemic hypersensitivity reaction

e) What kind of hypersensitivity reactions occur to latex? (2 marks)
- Type 1 hypersensitivity reaction: antigen and IgE. Systemic and immediate reaction
- Type 4 hypersensitivity reaction: antigen and T cell. Reaction takes up to 24 hours.
- Non-immune mediated reaction

f) List 4 groups that are at increased risk of latex allergy? (4 marks)
- Atopic patients
- Multiple surgical procedures in childhood
- Healthcare workers or other people with occupational exposure
- Allergy to bananas, chestnuts or avocado
- Patients who have required long term indwelling urinary catheters

4. Anaesthetic emergency II

Questions

It is a Saturday and you are anaesthetising emergency cases in theatre. You induce a 19-year-old man with no past medical history who has had an uneventful GA in the past, in the anaesthetic room without incident. You use a modified rapid sequence induction (propofol and suxamethonium) and then commence ventilation with sevoflurane for maintenance.

When you transfer him to theatre and connect him to monitoring you notice that his end-tidal carbon dioxide concentration is 7kPa, his heart rate is 120bpm, he is sweating profusely and his left arm (the arm with his cannula present in it) is hypertonic.

a) What do you think the most likely diagnosis is and list 2 other differentials? (3 marks)
b) List five other clinical features of the most likely diagnosis. (5 marks)
c) The end tidal carbon dioxide concentration increases to 22kPa, his core temperature measures 39.9°C and his heart rate is 180 beats per minute (bpm). What is your immediate management? (8 marks)
d) The patient's condition improves with your initial management. What would you do next? (4 marks)

Answers

a) What do you think the most likely diagnosis is and list 2 other differentials? (3 marks)
- Malignant hyperthermia is the most likely diagnosis
- Sepsis
- Inadequate ventilation and anaesthesia
- Thyroid storm
- Phaeochromocytoma

b) List five other clinical features of the most likely diagnosis. (5 marks)
- Early
  - **Metabolic**: increased oxygen consumption, mixed respiratory and metabolic acidosis, mottled skin
  - **Cardiovascular**: tachycardia, labile blood pressure
  - **Musculoskeletal**: masseter spasm, generalised muscle rigidity
- Late
  - **Metabolic**: hyperkalaemia, myoglobinuria, raised serum creatine kinase (CK), hyperthermia
  - **Cardiovascular**: arrhythmias, may lead to cardiac arrest
  - Disseminated intravascular coagulation

c) The end tidal carbon dioxide concentration increases to 22kPa, his core temperature measures 39.9°C and his heart rate is 180bpm. What is your immediate management? (8 marks)
- Stop trigger agent(s)
- Give 100% oxygen and hyperventilate
- Declare a critical incident and call for help. Inform the surgeons and postpone surgery
- Maintain anaesthesia using intravenous agents
- Muscle relaxation with non-depolarising agent (if necessary)
- Use a vapour free anaesthetic machine (can use Mapleson C circuit and oxygen cylinder until it is located)
- Continuous monitoring: $ETCO_2$, SpO_2, ECG, BP (preferably invasive), CVP
- Intravenous fluids
- Active cooling
- Dantrolene 2.5mg/kg initially followed by 1mg/kg bolus up to 10mg/kg
- Invasive lines (arterial line – measure blood gases: metabolic state, PaO_2 and $PaCO_2$, K^+. Insert central venous catheter and urinary catheter)
- Send formal bloods: CK, K^+, serum and urinary myoglobin, U&Es and coagulation profile
- Treat complications:
  - hyperkalaemia – insulin and dextrose and calcium chloride
  - arrhythmias – beta blockers, amiodarone, magnesium
  - acidosis – hyperventilation and sodium bicarbonate
  - myoglobinaemia – forced alkaline diuresis
  - DIC – fresh frozen plasma, cryoprecipitate and platelets

d) The patient's condition improves with your initial management. What would you do next? (4 marks)
- ITU admission for monitoring and further management
- Will still need surgery when stable
- Monitoring for relapse and need for further dantrolene

- Monitor renal function: may need renal replacement therapy
- Monitor for compartment syndrome
- Repeat and monitor creatine kinase (CK)
- Counsel patient and family
- Consider differential diagnoses and exclude when possible
- Refer to MH (malignant Hyperthermia) unit, Leeds

5. Major trauma

Questions

You are called to the emergency department as part of the trauma team. A 20-year-old male is *en route* with a suspected head injury having been involved in a road traffic accident and the estimated time of arrival (ETA) is 5 minutes. His GCS is reported as 10/15 at the scene of the accident.

a) What course of action will you take whilst awaiting the patient's arrival? (2 marks)

b) How would you assess this patient? (5 marks)

c) The patient's arterial blood gas shows a PaO_2 of 12kPa and $PaCO_2$ of 8.1kPa on 15 litres of oxygen. What course of action would you take? (2 marks)

d) What are the indications for intubating and ventilating patients with head injuries? (3 marks)

e) You intubate the patient successfully. What would you do next? (3 marks)

f) In the meantime, the patient becomes hypertensive and bradycardic. What is this response called and why does it occur? (2 marks)

g) What immediate treatment would you employ to treat this problem? (3 marks)

Answers

a) What course of action will you take whilst awaiting the patient's arrival? (2 marks)
- Attend the emergency department immediately and report to the trauma team leader
- Ensure airway/intubation equipment and drugs are prepared and in good working order
- Discuss the management plan with the trauma team leader and other members of staff

b) How would you assess this patient? (5 marks)
- I would undertake a full primary survey as per ATLS guidance
  - Airway (including C spine control).
    - Assess for airway patency and use jaw thrust if required. Apply oxygen and consider intubating (using manual inline stabilisation) if criteria for immediate intubation exist: GCS<8, loss of airway reflexes, inadequate ventilation or hypoxia
  - **Breathing**
    - Fully expose the chest looking for injuries (flail segments, penetrating injuries, bruising), asymmetry, respiratory rate and pattern. Palpate for crepitus and auscultate for bilateral air entry. Treat any life threatening injuries such as tension pneumothorax or sucking wounds. Take an arterial blood gas and put a pulse oximeter on
  - **Circulation**
    - Identify any sources of life threatening bleeding and control. Look at skin colour, feel temperature, capillary refill time and pulse. Control any other sources of bleeding. Secure IV access and take bloods; establish ECG and BP monitoring
  - **Disability**
    - Assess using **A**lert **V**oice **P**ain **U**nresponsive (AVPU) initially or GCS. Check pupillary sizes along with their response to light, and check blood sugar level. Assess pain at this point if appropriate
  - **Exposure**
    - Fully expose the patient looking for other injuries, not forgetting the back

c) The patient's arterial blood gas shows a PaO_2 of 12kPa and $PaCO_2$ of 8.1kPa on 15 litres of oxygen. What course of action would you take? (2 marks)
- Prepare to intubate and ventilate this patient, as his ventilation is inadequate in the presence of a suspected head injury
- Request another anaesthetist and experienced anaesthetic nurse or ODP to assist (potentially difficult airway, required to maintain manual in line stabilisation and need to ensure stable induction to prevent an increase in intracranial pressure (ICP) with laryngoscopy)
- Ensure all induction and emergency drugs are ready as well as intubation and difficult airway equipment

d) What are the indications for intubating and ventilating patients with head injuries? (3 marks)
- Airway – obstruction (blood or airway soiling), loss of laryngeal reflexes
- Breathing – hypoxia (PO_2<11KPa), hypercarbia (PCO_2 >6kPa), hypocarbia (PCO_2<4kPa)
- Disability – seizures, GCS<8, rapidly deteriorating GCS, pupillary signs or other focal neurology

e) You intubate the patient successfully. What would you do next? (3 marks)
- Ask another member of the trauma team to arrange an urgent CT of the patient's head and C-spine (and chest +/− abdomen if other serious injuries are suspected)
- Whilst waiting for the scan I would:
  - Airway: check that the airway is secured with tape not ties. Use a hard collar, blocks and tape to immobilise the C-spine

- Breathing: auscultate for air entry on both sides of the chest, insert an arterial line for beat-to-beat BP monitoring as well as for easy sampling of arterial blood gases. I would repeat the blood gas to ensure adequate ventilation (PO_2 >13kPa, PCO_2 4–5.5kPa)
- Circulation: insert 2 wide bore cannulae. Maintain MAP with fluids and vasopressor agents, as required
- Disability: ensure the patient is adequately sedated and paralysed to avoid coughing with consequent increased Intracranial pressure (ICP). Re-examine pupils. Position the patient with a 20° head-up tilt to reduce ICP, if thoracic and lumbar spine have been cleared (or tilt the whole trolley head-up if clearance is pending)
- Put the patient on a portable monitor (ECG, pulse oximeter, invasive BP). Ensure portable capnography is available. Check enough battery power on pumps used for sedation during transfer, and confirm adequate oxygen supply. Collect and check transfer bag, emergency drugs and portable suction

f) In the meantime, the patient becomes hypertensive and bradycardic. What is this response called and why does it occur? (2 marks)
  - It is a late physiological response (mediated by carotid body receptors) to a rise in ICP in an attempt to increase cerebral perfusion pressure. It is recognised by the triad of hypertension, bradycardia and an irregular breathing pattern

g) What immediate treatment would you employ to treat this problem? (3 marks)
  - Recognise that this is an emergency situation requiring urgent intervention, and inform appropriate colleagues (neurosurgeons, trauma team leader, ITU)
  - Ensure trolley 15–20° head-up, loosen collar around C-spine and ensure adequate venous drainage of the head and neck. Keep CVP low
  - Avoid hypoxia and hypercapnoea (keep $PaCO_2$ low-normal). No positive end-expiratory pressure(PEEP)
  - Ensure adequate sedation and muscle relaxation
  - Avoid drugs causing cerebral vasodilation
  - Osmotic +/− loop diuretics (mannitol 1g/kg +/− furosemide) or hypertonic saline

6. Displaced tracheostomy tube

Questions

You are called urgently to ITU to see a patient with a tracheostomy in situ who has desaturated after being turned. When you arrive you notice that the patient has a respiratory rate of 40 breaths per minute, oxygen saturations of 78% and he appears agitated.

a) How will you approach the patient? (5 marks)

Despite your interventions the patient becomes drowsy, his respiration becomes shallow and there is minimal movement of the bag with respiration or with assisted ventilation. His oxygen saturations remain around 80%. It becomes clear that the tracheostomy tube has become dislodged.

b) How will you proceed? (5 marks)
c) Your initial attempt at laryngoscopy reveals a grade 4 view. What would do before a further attempt at laryngoscopy? (3 marks)

Despite your interventions you are still unable to intubate the patient.
d) What would you do next? (2 marks)

After 2 intubation attempts you are struggling to ventilate the patient.
e) How would you manage this situation? (3 marks)

The ENT registrar arrives.
f) What will you ask him to do? (2 marks)

Answers

a) How will you approach the patient? (5 marks)
- In an ABC manner
- Ensure he is receiving 100% oxygen (check it's connected and being delivered)
- Check the tracheostomy tube – is the cuff inflated? Has it become dislodged (check capnograph)? Is there a speaking valve in place? Is there an inner tube that has become blocked?
- Suction
- Check the monitoring equipment (pulse oximeter – is it working?)
- Attach Mapleson C circuit with 100% oxygen
- Call for help – senior anaesthetist, ENT surgeon

Despite your interventions the patient becomes drowsy, his respiration becomes shallow and there is minimal movement of the bag with respiration or with assisted ventilation. His oxygen saturations remain around 80%. It becomes clear that the tracheostomy tube has become dislodged.

b) How will you proceed? (5 marks)
- Apply 100% via a face mask
- Try to replace the dislodged tracheostomy tube if more than 10 days old using a bougie and a tracheostomy tube of the same size as the original or one size smaller. If this is not possible, cover the tracheostomy site
- Prepare to intubate the patient if the above fails. Ensure there is a second anaesthetist to assist, that the difficult airway trolley is available and that all the intubation and emergency equipment/drugs are ready
- Discuss the plan with the nursing staff
- Find out vital information about the patient – previous laryngoscopy grade, reason for tracheostomy, past medical history. Ensure that the trachea can be accessed from the upper airway

On arrival of the second anaesthetist you begin inducing the patient, having confirmed that you can ventilate the patient using bag mask ventilation. The ENT registrar is *en route*.

c) Your initial attempt at laryngoscopy reveals a grade 4 view. What would do before a further attempt at laryngoscopy? (3 marks)
- Optimise head and neck position
- Move the pillow
- Suction airway if required
- Re-oxygenate and ventilate using BMV
- Reduce cricoid pressure
- Ensure bougie to hand
- Use a different laryngoscope blade or videolaryngoscope

Despite your interventions you are still unable to intubate the patient.

d) What would you do next? (2 marks)
- Return to bag mask ventilation (BMV)
- Call for more help – ENT, consultant

After 2 intubation attempts you are struggling to ventilate the patient.

e) How would you manage this situation? (3 marks)

Basic airway manoeuvres (head tilt, chin lift)

- 2-person technique for BMV
- Maximum head extension
- Verbalise "can't intubate can't ventilate"
- Oropharyngeal or nasopharyngeal airway
- 2 attempts at LMA insertion, return to BMV between each attempt

The ENT registrar arrives.

f) What will you ask him to do? (2 marks)

- Explain 'can't intubate, can't ventilate' scenario
  - Urgent siting of surgical airway or cricothyroidotomy is required

7. Collapse following epidural bolus

Questions

You are the anaesthetist on-call for labour ward. You are called urgently to review a 39-week primiparous woman who is in the second stage of labour. She had an epidural sited approximately 3 hours ago, which was working very well. The midwife claims the patient complained of 'weak arms' then became unresponsive following an epidural top-up given a few minutes ago.

a) What is your immediate management? (4 marks)

You identify the patient is not breathing and has a slow, low volume pulse.

b) How would you assist ventilation and assess its effectiveness? (4 marks)

c) How will you support the circulation? (3 marks)

A high epidural block or 'total spinal' is a possible cause for the patient's collapse.

d) Name three other differential diagnoses. (3 marks)

e) What else should be monitored? (1 mark)

f) In the event of ongoing cardiovascular and respiratory depression, what should be considered? (1 mark)

g) What is the maximum safe dose of bupivicaine? (1 mark)

h) In the event of cardiovascular collapse secondary to suspected local anaesthetic toxicity, what agent is indicated in addition to routine resuscitation? (1 mark)

i) What is the initial dose of this agent in a 70kg adult? (1 mark)

j) Is propofol a suitable substitute? (1 mark)

Answers

a) What is your immediate management? (4 marks)
- SAFE approach – Shout for help, Approach with care, Free from danger, Evaluate
- Call for help – senior obstetrician and senior anaesthetist at least
- Assess for signs of life – response to voice/stimulation, ABC approach – breathing and pulse check (10 seconds)
- If no signs of life or you are concerned the patient is 'peri-arrest' initiate a cardiac arrest call

You identify the patient is not breathing and has a slow, low volume pulse.

b) How would you assist ventilation and assess its effectiveness? (4 marks)
- Establish an airway – initially likely to be with an oropharyngeal airway and bag valve mask
- 100% oxygen
- Oxygen saturation monitoring
- Auscultate the chest
- Intubate as soon as possible (the patient is at high risk of aspiration)
- Arterial blood gas

c) How will you support the circulation? (3 marks)
- Position the patient in a left lateral tilt or displace the uterus manually to avoid aorto-caval compression
- Insert 2 large-bore IV cannulae
- Send blood for cross match, full blood count, coagulation screen, urea and electrolytes and glucose.
- Monitor blood pressure, heart rate and capillary refill time
- IV fluids
- Vasopressors if required. This is likely to require an arterial line and central venous line insertion at a later stage

A high epidural block or 'total spinal' is a possible cause for the patient's collapse.

d) Name three other differential diagnoses. (3 marks)
- Local anaesthetic toxicity (i.e. epidural catheter may have migrated into a blood vessel)
- Amniotic fluid embolism
- Pulmonary embolism
- Venous air embolism
- Occult haemorrhage (e.g. placental abruption)
- Intra-cerebral bleed
- Myocardial infarction
- Sepsis
- Anaphylaxis
- Acute exacerbation of asthma

e) What else should be monitored? (1 mark)
- The foetus, using CTG monitoring

f) In the event of ongoing cardiovascular and respiratory depression, what should be considered? (1 mark)
- Caesarean section
  - Delivery will be beneficial to maternal circulation and advantageous to the foetus if signs of foetal distress are evident

g) What is the maximum safe dose of bupivicaine? (1 mark)
- 2mg/kg

h) In the event of cardiovascular collapse secondary to suspected local anaesthetic toxicity, what agent is indicated in addition to routine resuscitation? (1 mark)
- 20% lipid emulsion (Intralipid®)

i) What is the initial dose of this agent in a 70kg adult? (1 mark)
- 1.5mls per kg (or 100ml) of 20% lipid emulsion, over 1 minute

j) Is propofol a suitable substitute? (1 mark)

- No

8. Defibrillation

Questions

You are the anaesthetic registrar on call when you receive a cardiac arrest call to one of the surgical wards. On your arrival, you see three nurses by the side of the bed of an elderly gentleman. One appears to be bag-mask ventilating the patient, the second is performing chest compressions and the third is wheeling in the cardiac arrest trolley. All say they have never managed a real cardiac arrest. None of the other resuscitation team members has arrived yet.

a) What are your first actions? (4 marks)
b) What is the correct positioning for defibrillation pads? (2 marks)
c) Is there any other way these can be applied? (2 marks)
d) The patient has a permanent pacemaker. Does this change anything? Why? (2 marks)

You see the rhythm shown in Figure 10.2 on the monitor.

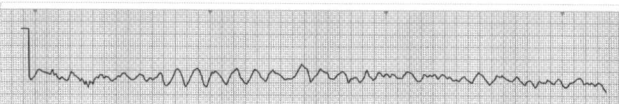

Figure 10.2 ECG

Courtesy of Dr Oliver Meyer

e) What is the rhythm? (1 mark)
f) How would you manage this patient? (4 marks)

On reassessment the rhythm shown in Figure 10.3 is seen.

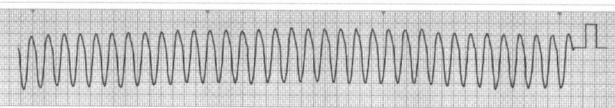

Figure 10.3 ECG

Courtesy of Dr Oliver Meyer

g) What rhythm is shown in Figure 10.3? (1 mark)
h) What would you do? (2 marks)

The patient was in hospital for treatment of small bowel obstruction.

i) Name two reversible causes for cardiac arrest which may be associated with small bowel obstruction and explain your reasons. (2 marks)

Answers

a) What are your first actions? (4 marks)
  - SAFE approach – Shout for help. Approach with care. Free from danger. Evaluate
  - Confirm cardiac arrest (response to voice/stimulation, breathing and pulse check for 10 seconds)
  - Commence / continue effective resuscitation according to the ALS algorithm
  - Connect the patient to cardiac monitor and assess rhythm
  - Attach defibrillation pads

b) What is the correct positioning for defibrillation pads? (2 marks)
  - To the right of the upper sternum, below the clavicle
  - 5th left intercostal space in the mid axillary line (V6 ECG electrode position)

c) Is there any other way these can be applied? (2 marks)
  - Antero-posterior placement
    - The anterior pad: left anterior chest, midway between the xiphoid process and the left nipple (corresponding to the V2–V3 ECG electrode position)
    - The posterior pad: beneath the left scapula

d) The patient has a permanent pacemaker. Does this change anything? Why? (2 marks)
  - The defibrillator pads should be placed 12–15cm from the pacemaker unit to minimise the risk of burns (the current from the defibrillator may travel along the pacemaker wire to the myocardium)
  - Antero-posterior pad placement can also be used

You see the rhythm shown in Figure 10.2 on the monitor.

e) What is the rhythm? (1 mark)
  - Ventricular fibrillation

f) How would you manage this patient? (4 marks)
  - A DC shock is indicated (150–200J on a biphasic machine)
  - CPR should continue (at a 30:2 ratio) until the shock is ready to be delivered
  - Immediately prior to delivering the shock the person delivering it should warn everyone to stand clear and, when safe to do so, shock the patient
  - CPR should recommence immediately for a further 2 minutes before reassessing
  - During this time reversible causes (4Hs and 4Ts) should be considered
  - Oxygen attached to a bag-valve-mask should be used for ventilation (30:2) and advanced airway management considered
  - Adrenaline 1mg IV every 3–5 minutes
  - IV access

On reassessment the rhythm shown in Figure 10.3 is seen.

g) What rhythm is shown in Figure 10.3? (1 mark)
  - Ventricular tachycardia

h) What would you do? (2 marks)
  - Confirm no pulse
  - Shock (150–360 J with a biphasic defibrillator)
  - Adrenaline 1mg intravenously after a third shock if required.
  - Amiodarone 300mg intravenously also following a third shock if required

The patient was in hospital for treatment of small bowel obstruction.

i) Name two reversible causes for cardiac arrest which may be precipitated by small bowel obstruction and explain your reasons. (2 marks)

- Aspiration leading to Hypoxia
- Vomiting leading to electrolyte disturbances (Hypo-/Hyper-kalaemia, -magnesaemia, -calcaemia)
- Hypovolaemia
- Prolonged immobility or underlying malignancy leading to thromboembolism

9. Reduced oxygen saturations in asthmatic patient following intubation

Questions

You are the anaesthetist for a gynaecology day surgery list. Your next patient has pelvic pain and is booked for a diagnostic laparoscopy. She has asthma, but no other medical problems and is appropriately fasted. You perform a routine induction with fentanyl and propofol, followed by atracurium to facilitate intubation. You see a grade 1 view at laryngoscopy, insert the tube uneventfully and tie it at 21cm at the lips.

You connect the oral endotracheal tube to the circle circuit and ventilator, and as you do so, you notice the oxygen saturation starts to drop suddenly on the monitor and the peak airway pressure is high.

a) What are your differential diagnoses? (4 marks)

b) What is your immediate management? (4 marks)

The oxygen saturation probe is giving a good trace on the monitor. The reading, though stable, is now 90% on 100% oxygen. The tube position is unchanged, but when you auscultate the chest you hear widespread wheeze and it is difficult to ventilate the patient. Other vital parameters are stable.

c) What will you do next? (4 marks)

d) If the patient fails to respond to these measures, what other treatment could you consider? (2 marks)

e) After initial resuscitation, what investigations may be useful? (2 marks)

f) What else will you need to think about? (2 marks)

You suspect this was an exacerbation of asthma.

g) Name two possible precipitants. (2 marks)

Answers

a) What are your differential diagnoses? (4 marks)
- Patient:
  - Acute exacerbation of asthma
  - Anaphylaxis
  - Tension pneumothorax
  - Aspiration
- Anaesthetic:
  - Endobronchial intubation
  - Insufficient relaxant dose
- Equipment:
  - Kinking or obstruction of circuit

b) What is your immediate management? (4 marks)
- Call for senior help
- 100% oxygen delivered with volatile (i.e. no air or nitrous oxide)
- Check pulse oximeter correctly attached
- Re-check oral endotracheal tube position ensuring cuff inflated and depth at lips unchanged
- Ventilate manually to assess ventilation
- Check for end-tidal carbon dioxide
- Look at chest expansion and auscultate lungs
- Check circuit for obstructions, blockages and faults
- Complete 'ABC' approach – check other vital parameters (ECG, heart rate, blood pressure, look for rash)

The oxygen saturation probe is giving a good trace on the monitor. The reading, though stable, is now 90% on 100% oxygen. The tube position is unchanged, but when you auscultate the chest you hear widespread wheeze and it is difficult to ventilate the patient. Other vital parameters are stable.

c) What will you do next? (4 marks)
- Maintain anaesthesia with a non-irritant, bronchodilating volatile, ideally sevoflurane
- Treat for an acute exacerbation of asthma in first instance, as most likely diagnosis
- In-line nebuliser or inhalers via endotracheal tube – salbutamol (2.5–5mg) + ipratropium bromide (500mcg)
- IV hydrocortisone 200mg
- IV magnesium 2g over approximately 15–20 minutes
- Discuss with the surgeon and consider postponing surgery

d) If the patient fails to respond to these measures, what other treatment could you consider? (2 marks)
- IV aminophylline
- IV salbutamol
- IV ketamine
- Worsening or severe refractory cases may require adrenaline

e) After initial resuscitation, what investigations may be useful? (2 marks)
- Chest X-ray
- Arterial blood gases (for monitoring progress)
- Serum tryptase if anaphylaxis suspected

f) What else will you need to think about? (2 marks)
- Electrolyte and fluid balance (beware of hypokalaemia with salbutamol)
- Inform ITU as the patient is likely to need ventilation, monitoring and careful extubation
- Patient will need to be informed afterwards
- Referral for allergy testing

g) You suspect this was an exacerbation of asthma. Name two possible precipitants. (2 marks)

- Atracurium
- Fentanyl

10. Intra-operative hypertension and tachycardia

Questions

You are anaesthetising an anxious 40-year-old gentleman for a para-umbilical hernia repair. He has a history of gastro-oesophageal reflux disease, so you decide to intubate him using a rapid sequence induction. The induction and transfer to theatre are uncomplicated. Starting blood pressure was 160/95mmHg, with a heart rate of 75bpm.

Approximately 15 minutes into the operation, you are writing the chart and suddenly the alarm sounds on the monitor. You look up and see the blood pressure is now 198/105mmHg and heart rate is 120bpm. The rhythm looks like a sinus tachycardia.

a) What is your immediate management? (2 marks)
b) List your differential diagnoses. (4 marks)
c) What specific interventions would you now undertake? (3 marks)
d) The patient remains hypertensive and tachycardic.
e) What will you do now? (2 marks)
f) Name 3 categories of drug that could be used to help reduce the blood pressure here and give examples. (3 marks)
g) What is sodium nitroprusside? How does it work? (2 marks)
h) Why is sodium nitroprusside infrequently used now? (1 mark)

You manage to reduce the blood pressure and heart rate of your patient and proceed with the procedure. However, towards the end of the operation, you notice ST segment depression on the ECG monitor.

i) What do you do? (3 marks)

Answers

(a) What is your immediate management? (2 marks)
- Check BP cuff and recycle the blood pressure to ensure correct reading, palpate pulse
- Increase FiO_2 to 100% (to help ensure maximum O_2 delivery to myocardium)
- Ask the surgeons to stop operating temporarily

(b) List your differential diagnoses (4 marks)
- Anaesthetic-related
  - Inadequate anaesthesia
  - Inadequate muscle relaxation
  - Hypercarbia secondary to re-breathing or inadequate ventilation
  - Drug administration, e.g. inadvertent adrenaline, ephedrine
- Surgical factors
  - Stress response
  - Painful stimulus
  - Drugs – e.g. administration of local anaesthetic with adrenaline
  - Bladder distension
- Patient-related
  - Uncontrolled hypertension (not taken medication)
  - Cardiac event
  - CNS/Autonomic reflexes triggered by surgery
  - Endocrine/Metabolic – phaeochromocytoma, thyroid storm

(c) What specific interventions would you now undertake? (3 marks)
- Deepen anaesthesia
- Analgesia
- Muscle relaxant (after ensuring the patient is adequately anaesthetised)
- Check circuit and ventilation to ensure normocarbia
- Rule out drug error or surgical drug administration
- Discuss degree of surgical stimulus with surgeons
- Venous blood gas to check electrolytes

The patient remains hypertensive and tachycardic.

(d) What will you do now? (2 marks)
- Call for senior help
- Inform surgeons about on-going clinical situation
- Consider pharmacological control of parameters

(e) Name 3 categories of drug that could be used to help reduce the blood pressure here and give examples (3 marks)
- Alpha$_1$-adrenoreceptor blockers – e.g. phentolamine (non-selective alpha-antagonist)
- Beta-adrenoreceptor blockers – e.g. labetalol (alpha and beta antagonist)
- Alpha$_2$-adrenoreceptor agonists – e.g. clonidine (reduced central sympathetic outflow)
- Direct vasodilators – e.g. glyceryl trinitrate (hypotensive action via nitric oxide. Useful if cardiac event suspected)

(f) What is sodium nitroprusside? How does it work? (2 marks)
- Direct vasodilator
- Its hypotensive action is mediated via nitric oxide

(g) Why is sodium nitroprusside infrequently used now? (1 mark)
  • Complex metabolism that produces free cyanide ions
  • These bind irreversibly to cytochrome oxidase and are potentially very toxic

You manage to reduce the blood pressure and heart rate of your patient and proceed with the procedure. However, towards the end of the operation, you notice ST segment depression on the ECG monitor.

(h) What do you do? (3 marks)
  • Indicates cardiac ischaemia. Increase oxygen delivery by increasing FiO_2
  • Maintain normotension (aiming for the patient's usual BP)
  • Ensure adequate analgesia
  • Consider low dose glyceryl trinitrate
  • Perform 12-lead ECG, blood tests (troponin, electrolytes, full blood count) and involve Cardiologist post-operatively
  • Discuss / inform senior anaesthetist

Pacemakers

Further reading

American College of Surgeons.*Advanced Trauma Life Support*, 2004

Association of Anaesthetists of Great Britain and Ireland, Malignant Hyperthermia Crisis Management, 2011. Available from: http://www.aagbi.org/sites/default/files/mh_guideline_for_website.pdf

Association of Anaesthetists of Great Britain and Ireland, Malignant Hyperthermia Crisis Task Allocations, 2011. Available from: http://www.aagbi.org/sites/default/files/MH_task_allocations_for_web.pdf

Association of Anaesthetists of Great Britain and Ireland, Management of a patient with suspected anaphylaxis during anaesthesia safety drill, 2009. Available from: http://www.aagbi.org/sites/default/files/ana_laminate_2009.pdf

Association of Anaesthetists of Great Britain and Ireland, Recommendations for the safe transfer of patients with brain injury, 2006. Available from: http://www.aagbi.org/sites/default/files/braininjury.pdf

Deakin C.*Clinical Notes for the FRCA*, Churchill Livingstone, 2011

Difficult Airway Society, Failed Intubation, Failed Ventilation, 2004. Available from: http://www.das.uk.com/guidelines/downloads.html

Mills A, Sice P, Ford S. Anaesthesia related anaphylaxis: investigation and follow-up. *Contin Educ Anaesth Crit Care Pain*, 14 (2): 57–62, 2014

Moppet I. Traumatic Brain Injury: assessment, resuscitation and early management. *Brit J Anaes*, 9 9 (1): 18–31, 2007

Regan K, Hunt K. Tracheostomy Management. *Contin Educ Anaesth Crit Care Pain*, 8 (1): 31–5, 2008

Resuscitation Council (UK), Resuscitation Guidelines 2016. Available from: http://www.resus.org.uk/pages/gl2010.pdf

Chapter 11 **Mock OSCE**

Introduction

This chapter includes a question for each station of the OSCE. It has been designed for practising all the skills learnt through out the rest of the book before checking through the answers.

1. Anatomy

Questions

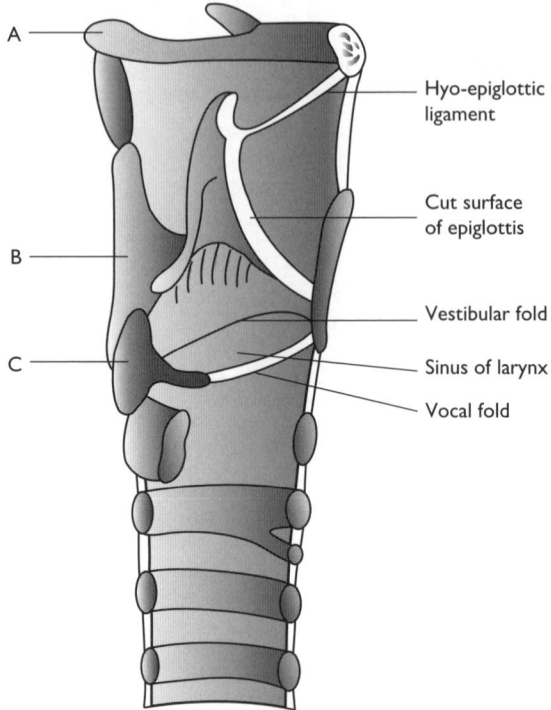

Figure 11.1 Anatomy of the larynx

Reproduced from Spoors, C and Kiff, K, Training in Anaesthesia, 2010 with permission from Oxford University Press

a) Identify structure A. (1 mark)
b) Identify structure B. (1 mark)
c) Identify structure C. (1 mark)
d) What is the role of the intrinsic muscles of the larynx? (1 mark)
e) Which muscle pair abducts the vocal cords? Describe how it achieves this. (2 marks)
f) What is the role of the extrinsic muscles of the larynx? (1 mark)
g) Which muscles elevate the larynx in the neck? (4 marks)
h) Which muscles depress the larynx? (3 marks)
i) Outline the motor supply to the intrinsic muscles of the larynx. (2 marks)
j) Outline the sensory nerve supply of the larynx. (2 marks)
k) What is the arterial blood supply of the larynx? (2 marks)

2. Technical Skills

Questions

a) Name 4 things you would like to check prior to performing a tracheostomy change. (4 marks)

b) What equipment will you assemble prior to starting the tracheostomy change? (4 marks)

c) Document 6 steps you would take during the process of changing the tracheostomy. (6 marks)

d) How would you confirm correct positioning of the new tube? (4 marks)

e) Name 2 complications that can occur when changing a tracheostomy tube. (2 marks)

3. History

Questions

You are asked to take an anaesthetic history from a 42-year-old lady having a hysterectomy.

a) You find out this lady is having a hysterectomy for menorrhagia due to fibroids, what do you want to ask now? (2 marks)

b) She tells you she has always been anaemic because she has thalassaemia. What do you want to ask now? (3 marks)

c) You move on to her past medical history – what further questions will you ask in a systems review? (6 marks)

d) You find out she has recently lost weight and been having night sweats, what else do you need to ask about? (6 marks)

e) How do conclude the interview? (3 marks)

4. Communication

Questions

This is Mrs Green, she is a primigravid woman in early labour. You are the labour ward anaesthetist and are asked to discuss an epidural with her.

a) How would you start the consultation? (2 marks)

b) She says that she is in pain and wants an epidural but doesn't know if she has any other options. (4 marks)

c) She says that she has tried pethidine and TENS and that they haven't worked. She thinks that she wants an epidural but is concerned about the side effects for her baby. (4 marks)

d) She has read that a woman was paralysed after an epidural and wants to know that this will not happen to her. (4 marks)

e) Her birthing plan stipulates that she wants to be active and be able to move around the room throughout labour. What would you discuss in relation to this? (3 marks)

f) She decides that she wants to go ahead with an epidural but asks if there are any other side effects that haven't been mentioned. (3 marks)

g) How would you finish your discussion? (1 mark)

5. Examination

Questions

Mrs Williams is thirty weeks pregnant and is listed for an elective caesarean section at thirty-nine weeks' gestation as she has had two previous sections. This is her pre-operative assessment visit. Please examine her.

a) How would you start the consultation? (1 mark)

b) How would you assess her airway? (3 marks)

c) Her BMI is 38. Apart from her airway what else would you like to assess? (3 mark)

d) She states that she has had some visual disturbance over the last week. What would you examine now? (6 marks)

e) What investigations would you like to request? (4 marks)

f) What is the definition of pre-eclampsia? (1 mark)

g) Why might regional anaesthesia be problematic in a patient with pre-eclampsia? (2 marks)

6. Radiology

Questions

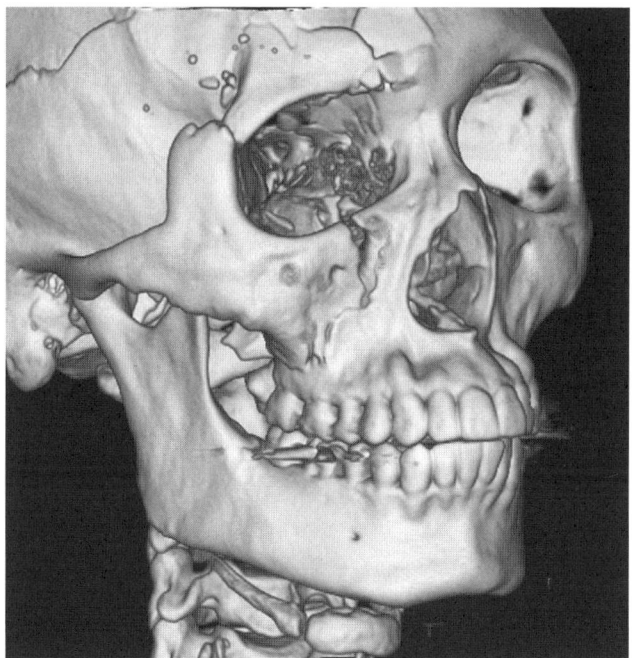

Figure 11.2 CT reconstruction

Look at Figure 11.2, are the following true or false?
a) There is frontal bone involvement in this injury. (1 mark)
b) The patient may have difficulty look inferiorly. (1 mark)
c) This represents a pure Le Fort II fracture. (1 mark)
d) This patient is at high risk of having a base of skull fracture. (1 mark)
e) This patient has a mandibular fracture. (1 mark)
f) The most common site for mandibular fractures is at the angle of the jaw. (1 mark)
g) Nasal intubation would be the most appropriate method of intubation for this patient in an emergency. (1 mark)
h) Maxillary fractures carry a high risk of significant bleeding. (1 mark)
i) Extubation is less problematic after fixation of maxillary fractures than after fixation of other facial fractures. (1 mark)
j) Radiation exposure for a CT head is equivalent to 2 years of background radiation exposure. (1 mark)

7. Equipment

Questions

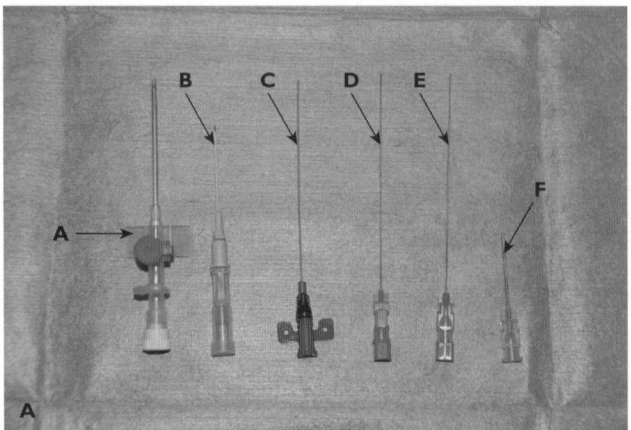

Figure 11.3a Needles and cannulas. Please see colour plate section.

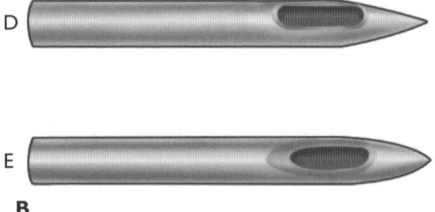

Figure 11.3b Spinal needle tips

Look at Figure 11.3a
a) Name the following types of cannulas and their gauges: A, B and C. (3 marks)
b) How is A sterilised? (1 mark)
c) What is the typical shelf life of A, as advised by the manufacturer? (1 mark)
d) What is different about C compared with the others? (1 mark)
e) Name 4 complications associated with inserting C. (4 marks)
f) What is the flow rate through a cannula directly proportional to? (2 marks)
g) What is the typical flow rate of water, in ml/min, through a 14G cannula? (2 marks)

Look again at Figures 11.3a and 11.3b
h) Name D and E. (2 marks)
i) What gauges of D are typically used in anaesthesia? (2 marks)
j) What is the purpose of F? (2 marks)

8. Hazards

Questions

a) What information regarding a pacemaker is required when planning elective surgery? (5 marks)

b) What do you understand by the term VVI pacemaker? (3 marks)

c) When is surgery considered high risk for pacemaker malfunction? (2 marks)

d) Which form of diathermy is preferably used when a pacemaker is present? (1 mark)

e) What general precautions should be taken when using all forms of diathermy in a patient with a pacemaker? (5 marks)

f) What specific precautions should be taken when using monopolar diathermy? (2 marks)

g) What should you ensure before starting elective surgery in a patient with an ICD? (2 marks)

9. Measurement and Monitoring

Questions

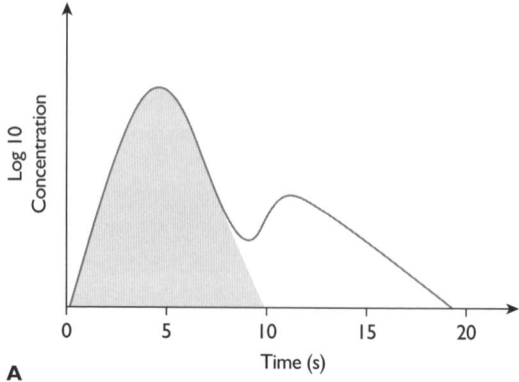

A

Figure 11.4a Thermodilution curve

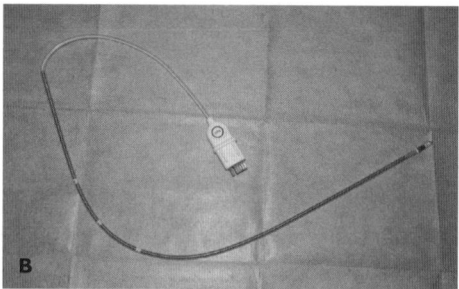

B

Figure 11.4b Probe. Please see colour plate section.

a) Use of the Fick principle to measure elimination of carbon dioxide is an example of which type of cardiac output measurement? (1 mark)

b) Complete the following equation, applying the Fick principle to the measurement of cardiac output:

Cardiac output = Rate of elimination of carbon dioxide from the lungs / (1 mark)

Look at Figure 11.4a. It shows a semi-logarithmic graph of washout curves for a dye dilution technique used to measure cardiac output in two patients.

c) Which dye is commonly used in this method? (1 mark)

d) What are the advantages of using this dye? (2 marks)

e) How is the cardiac output calculated? (2 marks)

f) Name an alternative dilution technique to dye? (1 mark)

g) What indwelling equipment is required to perform this? (1 mark)

h) What is injected down the line? (1 mark)

i) Where should the distal end of the channel used for injection lie? (1 mark)

j) Name two complications of using this line. (2 marks)

Look at Figure 11.4b

k) Identify the equipment in Figure 11.4b. (1 mark)

l) What does the probe measure? (1 mark)

m) How is this used to calculate cardiac output? (2 marks)

n) Where is the ideal probe tip location? (1 mark)

o) Name two advantages of this technique over other methods of cardiac output monitoring. (2 marks)

10. Resuscitation and Simulation

Questions

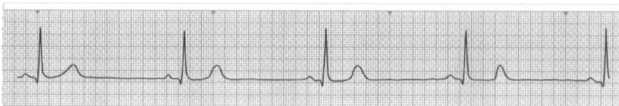

Figure 11.5 ECG

Courtesy of Dr Oliver Meyer

You are anaesthetising a 55-year-old obese woman for a laparoscopic cholecystectomy. The induction and intubation was uneventful and you are now in theatre, with a haemodynamically stable patient who is attached to the ventilator. The abdomen has been insufflated for 10 minutes.

You have been documenting the heart rate as 75–90bpm. The monitor suddenly alarms, and when you look up, the ECG shows a heart rate of 35bpm. The ECG complexes appear altered.

a) How will you manage this situation? (4 marks)
   When you palpate the carotid there is no pulse.

b) What will you do now? (4 marks)
   The cardiac arrest trolley arrives.

c) What will you do next? (2 marks)

You see Figure 11.5 on the defibrillator monitor, with the absence of a central pulse.

d) Look at Figure 11.5. Name and define this rhythm? (2 marks)

e) How will you manage this? (3 marks)

f) Would you give atropine? (1 mark)

g) List 4 of the possible reversible causes of this arrest? (2 marks)

h) What is the recommended maximum intra-peritoneal pressure during laparoscopic surgery?
   (1 mark)

i) What intra-peritoneal gas volume typically keeps the pressure below the recommended
   maximum? (1 mark)

1. Anatomy

Answers

a) Identify structure A. (1 mark)
- Hyoid bone

b) Identify structure B. (1 mark)
- Thyroid cartilage

c) Identify structure C. (1 mark)
- Arytenoid cartilage

d) What is the role of the intrinsic muscles of the larynx? (1 mark)
- To control the position of the vocal cords

e) Which muscle pair abducts the vocal cords? Describe how it achieves this. (2 marks)
- The posterior cricoarytenoid muscles rotate the arytenoid cartilages laterally

f) What is the role of the extrinsic muscles of the larynx? (1 mark)
- To control the position of the larynx in the neck; for example, during swallowing

g) Which muscles elevate the larynx in the neck? (4 marks)
- Digastric
- Myohyoid
- Geniohyooid
- Stylohyoid

NB. 3 other pairs of muscles provide supplemental function to elevate the larynx (thyrohyoid, hyoglossus, genioglossus).

h) Which muscles depress the larynx? (3 marks)

3 paired muscles:
- A – sternothyroid
- B – sternohyoid
- C – omohyoid

i) Outline the motor supply to the intrinsic muscles of the larynx. (2 marks)
- External branch of the superior laryngeal nerve supplies cricothyroid
- Recurrent laryngeal nerves supplies all of the intrinsic muscles with the exception of cricothyroid

j) Outline the sensory nerve supply of the larynx. (2 marks)
- Recurrent laryngeal nerves supplies sensation to the trachea and glottis below the level of the vocal cords
- Internal branch of the superior laryngeal nerve supplies sensation to the glottis above the vocal cords

k) What is the arterial blood supply of the larynx? (2 marks)

Branches of:
- Superior thyroid arteries
- Inferior thyroid arteries

2. **Technical Skills**

Answers

a) Name four things you would like to check prior to performing a tracheostomy change. (4 marks)

Any 4 of:
- When the tracheostomy was performed and if there were any difficulties with the procedure
- What grade of view was seen at the most recent laryngoscopy
- What FiO_2 the patient is currently receiving and the current ventilator settings
- The results of the most recent arterial blood gas
- When the NG feed was stopped

b) What equipment will you assemble prior to starting the tracheostomy change? (4 marks)
- Alternative means of oxygenation and ventilation (Facemask, orophayngeal airway, catheter mount, Mapleson C circuit or self-inflating bag)
- Occlusive dressing to cover the tracheostomy site in the event of needing to use an alternative means of ventilation
- Equipment for orotracheal intubation (laryngoscope, checked endotracheal tube)
- Equipment for tracheostomy change (suction catheter, bougie, airway exchange catheter, new tracheostomy tube, lubricant, syringe)

c) Document 6 steps you would take during the process of changing the tracheostomy. (6 marks)

Any 6 of:
- Establish monitoring – ECG, pulse oximetry, noninvasive blood pressure (NIBP), $EtCO_2$
- Position patient with neck extended
- Suction oropharynx and trachea (via tracheostomy)
- Check and prepare a new tube including checking and lubricating the cuff
- Insert suction catheter/bougie/airway exchange catheter through the existing tracheostomy
- Remove tube and railroad new tube over exchange device
- Inflate the cuff and hand ventilate the patient

d) How would you confirm correct positioning of the new tube? (4 marks)

Any 4 of:
- Hand ventilate the patient
- Check for chest wall movement
- Auscultate the chest
- End-tidal CO_2
- Fibre optic scope

e) Name 2 complications that can occur when changing a tracheostomy tube. (2 marks)
- Creation of a false passage
- Failure to reinsert tube

3. History

Answers

a) You find out this lady is having a hysterectomy for menorrhagia due to fibroids, what do you want to ask now? (2 marks)
- Has she been told she is anaemic?
- Is she on any treatment for this?
- Does she ever get any symptoms of lethargy, shortness of breath or chest pain?
- What is her exercise tolerance?

b) She tells you she has always been anaemic because she has thalassaemia. What do you want to ask now? (3 marks)
- Have you ever needed treatment for this?
- Have you ever required any blood transfusions?
- Does she know if she has sickle cell disease?

Thalassaemias are blood disorders leading to varying degrees of anaemia, from mild-moderate in those with α thalassaemias, to being transfusion-dependent in patients with β thalassaemias. They occur due to the absence of or the defective synthesis of the haemoglobin chains. Thalassaemia is more common in those of Mediterranean, Asian or African origin. Additionally, thalassamemia and sickle cell disease can co-exist so you should enquire as to her sickle cell status.

c) You move on to her past medical history – what further questions will you ask in a systems review? (6 marks)
- Any recent illnesses or injury, any previous admissions to hospital, and visits to the GP?
- Do you have diabetes, high blood pressure, heart disease, strokes, blood clots, asthma, COPD, epilepsy, and have you ever been jaundiced or had stomach ulcers?
- Then a systems review should include:
  - CVS: Chest pain/dyspnoea/palpitations/syncope/pre-syncope/ankle swelling/orthopnoea/PND
  - RS: Cough/dyspnoea/fever/night sweats
  - CNS: Headaches/dizziness/'funny turns'
  - GI: Anorexia/weight loss/N&V/GORD/change in bowel habit

d) You find out she has recently lost weight and been having night sweats, what else do you need to ask about? (6 marks)
- This clearly raises the suspicion of an underlying pathology. This may be an infectious disease such as malaria or TB, a chronic inflammatory process such as endocarditis, or it could be an underlying malignancy such as a lymphoma. Some pertinent questions include:
- For how long has this been going on?
- Have you previously sought medical attention for this – for example from your GP?
- Have you had any recent travel?
- Has anyone in your family/close friends or people you live with/have travelled with had similar symptoms?
- Has anybody she knows been diagnosed with TB?
- Has she noticed any lumps or bumps recently?

e) How do conclude the interview? (3 marks)
- Ask all the normal questions for surgical, drug, social and dental history
- Ask the patient if she has any concerns or further questions.
- Thank her and mention you will be speaking to a consultant about a few points that have been raised and that you will come back to talk with her about her management plan shortly

4. Communication

Answers

a) How would you start the consultation? (2 marks)
  - Introduce yourself and explain that you are the anaesthetist covering labour ward
  - Prompt the patient by saying that you understand she is considering an epidural

b) She says that she is in pain and wants an epidural but doesn't know if she has any other options. (4 marks)
  - Be empathetic towards her and reassure her that there are several options for managing her pain.
  - Ask what she has tried so far and if it has helped.
  - You will want to discuss:
    - oral analgesics
    - pethidine or diamorphine (in labour, usually given IM by midwives)
    - remifentanil patient controlled analgesia (PCA)
    - epidural analgesia
    - alternative therapies available such as hypnobirthing, water baths and transcutaneous electrical nerve stimulation (TENS)
  - It is worth checking that she hasn't got any medical or obstetric problems that would be a contraindication to any of these options

c) She says that she has tried pethidine and TENS and that they haven't worked. She thinks that she wants an epidural but is concerned about the side effects for her baby. (4 marks)
  - It is best to ask the patient what her particular concerns are. She may have preconceptions that are incorrect, or need further explanation of the side effects
  - Reassure her that epidurals are used frequently for women in labour with no detrimental effects on their babies
  - Explain clearly that there are a number of side effects that are very common, such as itching, leg weakness, shivering and a drop in blood pressure
  - Reassure her that she will be carefully monitored and will have a drip so that additional medication or fluids can be given very quickly if necessary

d) She has read that a woman was paralysed after an epidural and wants to know that this will not happen to her. (4 marks)
  - Do not be tempted to lie and say that there is no way that this could happen
  - Say that unfortunately there are some rare complications associated with epidurals. Explain that because the epidural sits near the spine and nerves these can occasionally get bruised
  - This would manifest as a patch of numbness or weakness that lasted after the epidural wore off and this happens in about 1:5,000 cases. This normally resolves completely within a few days or weeks, however, in a tiny proportion it can be a permanent numbness or weakness and this occurs in about 1:20,000 cases
  - A catastrophic complication, such as paralysis, could happen but is even more rare and is very unlikely in a young woman with no medical problems

e) Her birthing plan stipulates that she wants to be active and be able to move around the room throughout labour. What would you discuss in relation to this? (3 marks)
  - Make sure that she is aware that an epidural is likely to produce a certain degree of leg weakness and that she will have a drip and the epidural catheter attached to her which may hamper movement

- It might be best to offer to discuss this with the midwife so that a joint plan can be devised
- Warn her that she may be at risk of falling and that she should not attempt to move out of bed on her own

f) She decides that she wants to go ahead with an epidural but asks if there are any other side effects that haven't been mentioned. (3 marks)

- It is worth mentioning the risk of post dural puncture headache (around 1:100) and explaining that there are options to deal with this if it does occur
- Sometimes the epidural doesn't work completely and so may need to be re-sited
- You should also mention the possibility that epidurals can prolong labour and that there is an increased chance of needing an instrumental delivery because the abdominal muscles are weakened
- It is good to finish on a more positive note and say that there is no evidence to suggest that epidurals increase the chance of needing a caesarean section and that although a small amount of bruising of the back is normal, epidurals are not associated with long term back pain

g) How would you finish your discussion? (1 mark)

- Check that she has understood the information that you have given and ask if she has any further questions. It may be worth offering an information leaflet and time to reflect before making a final decision

5. Examination

Answers

Mrs Williams is thirty weeks pregnant and is listed for an elective caesarean section at thirty-nine weeks' gestation as she has had two previous sections. This is her pre-operative assessment visit. Please examine her.

a) How would you start the consultation? (1 mark)
- Introduce yourself and explain that you are going to perform an examination to help plan your anaesthetic

b) How would you assess her airway? (3 marks)
- Start with inspection and look for any features that might predict a difficult intubation such as a receding jaw, short neck, obesity, large amount of breast tissue, microstomia or signs of congenital disease that may affect intubation
- Ask her to open her mouth – assess her Mallampati score, mouth opening and dentition
- Ask her to extend her neck – assess her thyromental and sternomental distances

c) Her BMI is 38. Apart from her airway what else would you like to assess?
(3 mark)
- Examine her hands for signs of potential difficulties with intravenous access
- Examine her lumbar spine. Look for any deformities and ask her to sit in a similar position to that which you would require to actually site a spinal or epidural
- Palpate her iliac crests and spinous processes. Even in obese people, finding the landmarks is often not difficult

d) She states that she has had some visual disturbance over the last week. What would you examine now? (6 marks)
- Assess her for signs of pre-eclampsia
- Measure her blood pressure
- Look for ankle and sacral oedema
- Elicit reflexes in her lower limbs looking for hyperreflexia and clonus
- Examine her abdomen for any epigastric pain (a symptom of pre-eclampsia) or right upper quadrant pain (a sign of liver involvement)
- Offer to perform fundoscopy to rule out papilloedema
- Offer to examine her cranial nerves to rule out other causes of visual disturbance

e) What investigations would you like to request? (4 marks)
- A urine dipstick test for proteinuria. If there is greater than 1+ of protein further tests should be performed.
- A urinary protein:creatinine ratio of >30mg/mmol or a 24hr urinary collection with protein of >300mg indicates significant proteinuria Liver function tests – to measure transaminase and bilirubin levels and rule out Haemolysis, Elevated Liver enzymes, Low Platelets (HELLP) syndrome
- Renal function, urate and electrolytes
- A full blood count – to check platelet count
- A fetal ultrasound to assess fetal growth and umbilical vessel Doppler flow
- A CTG might be appropriate

f) What is the definition of pre-eclampsia? (1 mark)
- A new presentation of hypertension (>140/90 mmHg) after 20 weeks' gestation with significant proteinuria (>300mg in a 24hour period)

g) Why might regional anaesthesia be problematic in a patient with pre-eclampsia? (2 marks)
- The patient may have a low platelet count or be coagulopathic if there is liver involvement, and this increases the risk of a vertebral canal haematoma with regional anaesthesia
- In pre-eclampsia the patient is peripherally vasoconstricted but intravascularly deplete. Theoretically therefore, there is a risk of abrupt hypotension after spinal anaesthesia

6. Radiology

Answers

Look at Figure 11.2

a) There is frontal bone involvement in this injury. (1 mark)
- True
- There is a complex fracture involving the frontal bone

b) The patient may have difficulty look inferiorly. (1 mark)
- True
- The fracture passes through the inferior orbit and there may be entrapment of the interior rectus or inferior oblique muscles

c) This represents a pure Le Fort II fracture. (1 mark)
- False
- A pure Le Fort II fracture involves a pyramidal section of the midface becoming disrupted, with the apex at the naso-maxillary suture and the base involving the teeth. Here a zygomatic arch fracture is also present

d) This patient is at high risk of having a base of skull fracture. (1 mark)
- True
- Zygomatic fractures and Le Fort III fractures have the highest risk of associated base of skull fractures. Frontal fractures involving the sinuses can also cause dural tears

e) This patient has a mandibular fracture. (1 mark)
- False

f) The most common site for mandibular fractures is at the angle of the jaw. (1 mark)
- False
- The majority of mandibular fractures occur along the neck of the mandible

g) Nasal intubation would be the most appropriate method of intubation for this patient in an emergency. (1 mark)
- False
- In an emergency situation, securing the airway via the oral route may be most appropriate. For surgical fixation of maxillary and facial fractures, surgeons may request nasal intubation. This should only be done if a base of skull fracture has been ruled out

h) Maxillary fractures carry a high risk of significant bleeding. (1 mark)
- True
- Blood loss from maxillary fractures can be severe and should be considered as a major source of haemorrhage

i) Extubation is less problematic after fixation of maxillary fractures than after fixation of other facial fractures. (1 mark)
- False
- Oedema may compromise the airway for up to 48 hours after surgery

j) Radiation exposure for a CT head is equivalent to 2 years of background radiation exposure. (1 mark)
- False
- A CT head is equivalent to seven months of background exposure

7. Equipment

Answers

Look at Figure 11.3a

a) Name the following types of cannulas and their gauges: (3 marks)

- A – Orange 14G BD venflon
- B – Pink 20G Abbocath
- C – 20G Vygon arterial cannula (Seldinger)

b) How is A sterilised? (1 mark)

- Irradiation

c) What is the typical shelf life of A, as advised by the manufacturer? (1 mark)

- Three years

d) What is different about C compared with the others? (1 mark)

- Should be inserted into an artery (abbocaths are acceptable for venous cannulation)
- Inserted using a wire – Seldinger technique
- Is designed to be sutured into place

e) Name 4 complications associated with inserting C. (4 marks)

- Immediate:
  - Haemorrhage
  - Damage to surrounding structures – tissue, nerves (pain), veins
  - Wrong position of needle or cannula / failure of technique
- Delayed:
  - Fistula or aneurysm formation
  - Thrombus formation +/− embolism
  - Arterial occlusion and distal ischaemia
  - Infection
- Iatrogenic:
  - Erroneous drug administration through arterial cannula

f) What is the flow rate through a cannula directly proportional to? (2 marks)

- The pressure gradient across the cannula
- The diameter/radius of the cannula

g) What is the typical flow rate of water, in ml/min, through a 14G cannula? (2 marks)

- 14G = 250–360mL/min (270 mL/min specified on product page)

  Others:
  - 16G = 130–240mL/min (236 specified on product page)
  - 18G = 75–120mL/min (103 mL/min specified on product page)
  - 20G = 40–80mL/min (67 mL/min specified on product page)

Look again at Figures 11.3a and 11.3b

h) Name D and E. (2 marks)

- D – Whitacre spinal needle
- E – Sprotte spinal needle

i) What gauges of D are typically used in anaesthesia? (2 marks)

- 25G and 27G

j) What is the purpose of F? (2 marks)

- Spinal needle introducer
- Assists passage of spinal needle through skin, subcutaneous tissues and ligaments – reduces debris entering the needle and helps to stabilise and maintain the needle's shape

8. Hazards

Answers

a) What information regarding a pacemaker is required when planning elective surgery? (5 marks)
- When the device was last checked (should be within 3 months)
- Indication for device insertion
- Degree of pacemaker dependency
- Extent of heart failure
- If the device is approaching replacement date

b) What do you understand by the term VVI pacemaker? (3 marks)
- First letter indicates the chamber paced: atrium (A), ventricle (V), dual (D), none (O)
- Second letter indicates the chamber sensed: atrium (A), ventricle (V), dual (D), none (O)
- Third letter indicates response to sensing: triggered (T), inhibited (I), dual (D), none (O)
- Fourth letter indicates rate modulation or programmability: rate modulated (R), communicating (C), multi programmable (M), simple programmable (P), none (O)
- Fifth letter describes anti-tachycardia function: paced (P), shocks (S), dual (D)
- So VVI will pace the ventricle, sense the ventricle and respond by inhibiting it (i.e. if the ventricle stops contracting the pacemaker will pace at a set rhythm, stopping only when it senses a spontaneous ventricular contraction)

c) When is surgery considered high risk for pacemaker malfunction? (2 marks)
- Surgery site close to the implant
- Use of diathermy

d) Which form of diathermy is preferably used when a pacemaker is present? (1 mark)
- Bipolar

e) What general precautions should be taken when using all forms of diathermy in a patient with a pacemaker? (5 marks)
- Monitor ECG from before induction of anaesthesia
- Use an alternative method to detect pulse rather than ECG e.g. pulse oximeter, arterial line
- CPR and external pacing equipment immediately available
- Available cardiac technicians
- Ensure cables from/to the diathermy equipment are kept away from the site of the pacemaker

f) What specific precautions should be taken when using monopolar diathermy? (2 marks)
- Limit use to short bursts
- Ensure the return electrode is positioned so that the current pathway between the diathermy electrode and return electrode is as far away from the pacemaker as possible

g) What should you ensure before starting elective surgery in a patient with an ICD? (2 marks)
- ICD has been switched to a 'monitor only' mode to prevent inappropriate shocks
- There is easy access to the anterior chest wall, or defibrillator pads have been applied

9. Measurement and Monitoring

Answers

a) Use of the Fick principle to measure elimination of carbon dioxide is an example of which type of cardiac output measurement? (1 mark)
- Non invasive

b) Complete the following equation, applying the Fick principle to the measurement of cardiac output: (1 mark)
- Cardiac output = Rate of elimination of carbon dioxide from the lungs/venous concentration of CO_2 – arterial concentration of CO_2

Look at Figure 11.4a. It shows a semi-logarithmic graph of washout curves for a dye dilution technique used to measure cardiac output in two patients.

c) Which dye is commonly used in this method? (1 mark)
- Indocyanine green is used

d) What are the advantages of using this dye? (2 marks)
- Low toxicity
- Short half-life
- Favourable absorption characteristics – i.e. its absorption is unaffected my changes in oxygen saturation.

e) How is the cardiac output calculated? (2 marks)
- Cardiac output = Dose of dye injected / Area (shaded) under curve

f) Name an alternative dilution technique to dye? (1 mark)
- Thermal dilution

g) What indwelling equipment is required to perform this? (1 mark)
- A pulmonary artery catheter

h) What is injected down the line? (1 mark)
- 10mls of 5% dextrose at approximately $0^\circ C$

i) Where should the distal end of the channel used for injection lie? (1 mark)
- At the junction of the superior vena cava and right atrium

j) Name two complications of using this line. (2 marks)
- Complications associated with internal jugular cannulation e.g. damage to surrounding vessels/ nerves, bleeding, infection etc.
- Complications from catheter passage through the heart e.g. arrhythmias, heart block, kinking, and valve damage
- Complications from presence in pulmonary artery e.g. arterial damage/rupture, thrombosis, pulmonary infarction

Look at Figure 11.4b
k) Identify the equipment in Figure 11.4b. (1 mark)
- Oesophageal Doppler probe

l) What does the probe measure? (1 mark)
- The velocity of blood in the descending thoracic aorta

m) How is this used to calculate cardiac output? (2 marks)
- Velocity of blood in the descending thoracic aorta is used to estimate the length of a column of blood passing through the aorta per unit time

- This is multiplied by the cross-sectional area (calculated based on age, sex, height and weight) of the aorta to give stroke volume
- Cardiac output = heart rate x stroke volume

n) Where is the ideal probe tip location? (1 mark)

- Between the fifth and sixth thoracic vertebrae. At this point the descending aorta is adjacent to and parallel to the distal oesophagus

o) Name two advantages of this technique over other methods of cardiac output monitoring. (2 marks)

- Relatively safe, minimally invasive and simple to use/insert
- The smooth muscle tone of the oesophagus naturally maintains the position of the probe for repeated measurements
- The oesophagus is in close proximity to the aorta, so signal interference from bone, soft tissue and lung is minimised

10. Resuscitation and Simulation

Answers

a) How will you manage this situation? (4 marks)
- Airway, breathing, circulation (ABC) approach
- 100% oxygen, check oxygen saturations
- Switch to manual ventilation to check endotracheal tube and ventilation
- Palpate for central pulse (carotid easiest to access) and check BP
- Tell the surgeons to deflate abdomen
- Consider atropine or glycopyrrolate if the heart rate (HR) does not improve

When you palpate the carotid there is no pulse.

b) What will you do now? (4 marks)
- Call for senior help (emergency buzzer) and place cardiac arrest call (2222)
- Tell surgeons to stop operating and deflate abdomen
- Level the operating table and commence CPR in accordance with ALS guidelines
- Start chest compressions at rate of 100 per minute
- Patient is intubated so perform continuous chest compressions

The cardiac arrest trolley arrives.

c) What will you do next? (2 marks)
- Connect patient to defibrillator
- Stop and assess rhythm

You see Figure 11.5 on the defibrillator monitor, with the absence of a central pulse.

d) Look at Figure 11.5 Name and define this rhythm? (2 marks)
- Pulseless Electrical Activity
- Cardiac electrical activity that would be expected to produce a cardiac output in the absence of a palpable pulse

e) How will you manage this? (3 marks)
- Re-commence CPR (non-shockable rhythm)
- Reassess every 2 minutes
- IV adrenaline 1mg every 3–5 minutes
- Consider 4Hs and 4Ts

f) Would you give atropine? (1 mark)
- No longer recommended in the ALS guidelines, as no evidence of any benefit in cardiac arrest

g) List 4 of the possible reversible causes of this arrest? (2 marks)
- Thromboembolism
- Hypoxia
- Hypo-/hyperkalaemia
- Hypovolaemia
- Tension pneumothorax

h) What is the recommended maximum intra-peritoneal pressure during laparoscopic surgery? (1 mark)
- 20cm H_2O

i) What intra-peritoneal gas volume typically keeps the pressure below the recommended maximum? (1 mark)
- 3–5 litres

Further reading

Rosen C, Simpson C. *Operative techniques in laryngology*. Spinger, 2008

Intensive Care Society, Standards for the care of adult patients with a temporary tracheostomy, (ICS, 2008). http://www.ics.ac.uk/ics-homepage/guidelines-standards/

Medicines and Healthcare Products Regulatory Agency. Guidelines for the perioperative management of patients with implantable pacemakers or implantable cardioverter defibrillators, where the use of surgical diathermy is anticipated (MHRA, 2006). Available from http://www.mhra.gov.uk/home/groups/dts-bi/documents/websiteresources/con2023451.pdf

Hans GA, Jones N. Preoperative Anaemia. *Contin Educ Anaesth Crit Care Pain*, Oxford Journals, 2013

http://www.oaa-anaes.ac.uk/assets/_managed/editor/File/Info%20for%20Mothers/PR_leaflets/PAIN%20 RELIEF%20IN%20LABOUR_JULY%202013.pdf

http://www.oaa-anaes.ac.uk/assets/_managed/editor/File/Info%20for%20Mothers/EIC/2008_eic_english.pdf

Subject Index